UNIT 731

UNIT 731

LABORATORY OF THE DEVIL, AUSCHWITZ OF THE EAST

JAPANESE BIOLOGICAL WARFARE IN CHINA 1933–45

YAN-JUN YANG
YUE-HIM TAM

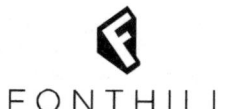

FONTHILL

First published in Great Britain in 2018 by Fonthill
An imprint of Pen & Sword Books Ltd
Yorkshire – Philadelphia
Reprinted 2021, 2026

ISBN 978-1-78155-678-8

The Publisher's authorised representative in the EU for product safety is
Authorised Rep Compliance Ltd., Ground Floor, 71 Lower Baggot Street, Dublin D02 P593, Ireland.
www.arccompliance.com

For a complete list of Pen & Sword titles please contact

PEN & SWORD BOOKS LIMITED
47 Church Street, Barnsley, South Yorkshire, S70 2AS, England
E-mail: enquiries@pen-and-sword.co.uk
Website: www.pen-and-sword.co.uk
or
PEN AND SWORD BOOKS
1950 Lawrence Road, Havertown, PA 19083, USA
E-mail: uspen-and-sword@casematepublishers.com
Website: www.penandswordbooks.com

Acknowledgements

The early parts of this book were initiated by Yan-jun Yang, professor in the Harbin Academy of Social Sciences and deputy curator of the Museum of the War Crimes by the Japanese Imperial Army Unit 731.

Yang, a specialist in details of the compound left by Unit 731, had studied the victimisation of live humans by Japanese scientists of the unit. He had been eager to put his research into proper historical context and to introduce his findings to the Western world for some time with little result.

In the summer of 2013, at the suggestion of Dr Don Tow, President of the New Jersey Alliance for Learning and Preserving the History of World War II in Asia, Yang invited Dr Yue-him Tam, Professor of History at Macalester College, St Paul, Minnesota, USA, to co-author a book. A specialist in Japanese Studies, Dr Tam is one of the very few scholars in the West to study and teach the history of Imperial Japan's war crimes in Asia during the Second World War and the memory issues in the post-war decades. Coincidentally, Dr Tam is Yang's long-time friend and mentor in the study of Sino-Japanese relations with special references to war crimes by Imperial Japan and issues of post-war remembrance.

Working closely together, Yang and Tam have expanded the historical perspectives of the book. As Dr Tam was responsible for rendering the text into English, he has sought editorial assistance from special readers: Mr Wilson Lee and Miss Yilin Wong, then PhD students in Japanese Studies at the Chinese University of Hong Kong, helped render technical Japanese terms into readable English, while breathing fresh air into the text from vantage points of the younger generation. The authors are also grateful to Ms Karin Winegar, a veteran freelance journalist and independent author based in St Paul, Minnesota, who helped make unprecedented gruesome issues of biochemical warfare easily understandable to Western readers. Ms Winegar also streamlined the narrative in English by clarifying technical and academic jargon.

The co-authors extend their special gratitude to the editors at Fonthill Media for their patience and understanding of our delay in submitting our manuscripts. We also take responsibility for any factual errors in the book. We are particularly moved by their endorsement of our belief that worldwide peace, justice, and prosperity will prevail and endure so long as nations shall do unto others as they would have others do unto them.

Contents

Introduction

During the Second World War, many heinous events took place. Some of those events affected international relations, some changed the fate of an entire people, while others caused crises upon all humankind or tremendous consequences upon future generations.

Although the war ended more than seventy years ago, the collective memory and the public history of this war haunt us today: in Poland, Auschwitz concentration camp lays bare the holocaust of the Jewish people by Germany's Nazis, while in Japan, Hiroshima Peace Memorial Park immortalises the epic tragedy of the first atomic bomb dropped by the United States in August 1945. Auschwitz and Hiroshima are globally significant historical sites, and thanks to these and other memorials, we are reminded that a nation that forgets the past is condemned to repeat the mistakes in the future.

Other war crimes of similar magnitude from that period have remained largely unexposed; this book aims to highlight the atrocities committed by the Japanese on China. The use of live human beings in biochemical experiments and the implementation of germ warfare by Japanese Imperial Army Unit 731 in China during the Second World War are rarely known outside China, particularly not in the Western world.

This book uncovers and details the scope and nature of inhumane and unethical acts by Japanese scientists under the direction of the Imperial Army of Japan in the massive compound called Unit 731 in Harbin, China. More than a million visitors annually come to this museum in Harbin to grieve, to learn, and to pay tribute to the victims and view its artefacts and documents.

The horrific legacy of Unit 731 and its relevant material should be preserved and recognised as significant 'Negative Heritage Properties', to remind the world of the importance of peace and the power of mass killing through biochemical war.

The authors uncover and expose the criminal activities of Unit 731 and their impacts both during the war and in the post-war years. Based on scholarly research, but framed in a style suitable for the general reader, the narrative includes a large number of photographs to illuminate points. We strongly believe in friendship with the people of Japan and those of Japanese descent, for they were also peace-loving and victims of Imperial Japan's militarism during the Second World War.

It is the authors' hope that readers share our respect for history and humanity, and that they support our conviction that only through historical truth can there be certain justice for victims, can humanity be safeguarded from repeating the mistakes of the past, and that genuine reconciliation and lasting peace among nations can be brought about.

Formation,
Expansion, and End of Unit 731

China and Japan are neighbouring East Asian countries, separated by a sea. Although both countries use Chinese characters (*Kanji*) that are almost indistinguishable to Europeans, gaps and misunderstandings have existed between China and Japan. They share the same cultural background historically, yet China and Japan have developed into states with different civilisations and customs.

Nevertheless, behind the differences, close connections remain between the two nations. As early as China's Tang dynasty (AD 618–907), China had been Japan's teacher. A Buddhist monk named Rev. Jianzhen (or Ganjin) attempted to visit Japan six times, eventually arriving there in AD 754. He brought important elements of rich Chinese civilisation and Buddhist culture to Japan that were immensely influential in the establishment of Japanese politics and culture. During the Ming dynasty (AD 1368–1644), however, Japan no longer regarded China as its teacher, and Japanese pirates looted coastal areas of China.

The powerful Industrial Revolution in Europe forced both China and Japan to enter the international community during the modern period, with Japan becoming China's teacher. After the 1853 arrival in Tokyo Bay of Commodore Matthew C. Perry of the United States Navy, Japan began to modernise. Following the Meiji Restoration of 1868, it developed into the most advanced nation in Asia, a paradigm of *Datsu-A Nyū-Oō*—leaving Asia and joining Europe. Following the development and expansion of international industrialisation, Japan caught the fast track and rose to become a world power. China, by comparison, despite having been the strongest country in the region for over a thousand years, became isolated, conservative, and declined.

It is difficult to maintain peace with one country strong and the other weak. Although China's Qing government sent a number of students to Japan to acquire political skill and technological expertise, China missed the best timing for reform, being at a disadvantage following a series of internal disunity and natural disasters against the imperial powers.

With the rise of national power and the spiritual influence of *bushidō*, Japan's desire for territorial expansion steadily strengthened: it invaded Taiwan in 1874; unleashed war with China in 1894; participated in the Eight-Nation Alliance to occupy China's capital, Beijing, in 1900; won the Russo-Japanese War in north-eastern China in 1905; and annexed the Korean Peninsula in 1910.

Within decades, Japan had hugely benefitted from war compensation and other diplomatic advantages because of victories in these external invasions, and this greatly aroused Japan's ambition to invade continental China. In 1927, the Cabinet of Japan suggested the Continental Policy: '... if we [Japan] want to conquer the world, we need to conquer China first. If we want to conquer China, we need to conquer Mongolia and Manchuria first. If we want to conquer Mongolia and Manchuria, we need to conquer Korea and Taiwan first'. This was later conceptualised as the 'Great East Asia Co-Prosperity Sphere'.

On 18 September 1931, Japan triggered the Manchurian Incident (known as the 'September 18 Incident' in Chinese), and within a few months, it occupied all of north-east China, a geographical area three times the size of Japan proper. Afterwards, Japan advocated the establishment of Manchukuo, allegedly ruled by the Chinese, but in reality a puppet state. Headed by Henry Puyi, the last Emperor of China, as the Chief Executive in 1932 and as Emperor in 1934, Manchukuo was actually controlled by Japanese, who determined every important issue.

With continuous external invasion and colonial expansion, militarism spread widely in Japan. In this context, Japan began to abrogate all international treaties, abandon morals and ethics, and devoted its efforts to research and manufacturing biochemical weapons of mass destruction in aggressive wars against neighbours in the Asian Pacific region. Consistent with this philosophy, Unit 731 of the Kwantung Army was formed.

Japan Violated International Treaties, Secretly Prepared and Executed Bacteriological Warfare

On 17 June 1925 in Geneva, Switzerland, thirty-seven countries, including Japan, the United States, and Germany, signed the 'Protocol for the Prohibition of the Use in War of Asphyxiating, Poisonous or other Gases, and of Bacteriological Methods of Warfare', commonly known as the Geneva Protocol.

The Protocol specifies:

Whereas the use in war of asphyxiating, poisonous or other gases, and of all analogous liquids, materials or devices, has been justly condemned by the general opinion of the civilized world; and Whereas the prohibition of such use has been declared in Treaties to which the majority of Powers of the world are Parties; and To the end that this prohibition shall be universally accepted as a part of International Law, binding alike the conscience and the practice of nations; Declare: That the High Contracting Parties, so far as they are not already Parties to Treaties prohibiting such use, accept this prohibition, agree to extend this prohibition to the use of bacteriological methods of warfare and agree to be bound as between themselves according to the terms of this declaration.[1]

The 'Convention on the Prohibition of the Development, Production and Stockpiling of Bacteriological (Biological) and Toxin Weapons and on their Destruction', which was opened for signature on 10 April 1972, addresses biological warfare similarly:

> Recognizing the important significance of the Protocol for the Prohibition of the Use in War of Asphyxiating, Poisonous or Other Gases, and of Bacteriological Methods of Warfare, signed at Geneva on 17 June 1925, and conscious also of the contribution which the said Protocol has already made and continues to make, to mitigating the horrors of war.[2]

Although the Japanese Government signed the Geneva Protocol in 1925, it never officially endorsed or abided by the Protocol. The Japanese military violated the international treaty by using chemical and bacteriological weapons in battlefields. According to Ji Xueren, a researcher from the Chemical Prevention Institute of the Chinese People's Liberation Army, 'from 1928 to 1945, the Japanese military committed the usage of chemical weapons 1,919 times in 20 provinces such as Heilongjiang, Jilin, Hebei, Shandong, Hunan and Henan'.[3]

Public information also reveals that the Japanese military committed large-scale usage of bacteriological weapons in Hohhot of Inner Mongolia, west Shandong, Changde of Hunan, Guangfeng and Shangrao of Shanxi, and Yiwu, Quzhou, Jinhua, and Ningbo of Zhejiang, causing death and injuries of a great number of innocent civilians, including women and children.

Interrogation of Shirō Ishii

On 6 February 1946, Lt-Gen. Shirō Ishii, the first commander of Unit 731, and Lt-Gen. Masaji Kitano, second commander of the Unit, were interrogated in Tokyo, Japan, by Lt-Col. Arvo T. Thompson from Fort Detrick, Frederick, Maryland. Ishii acknowledged Unit 731 committed bacteriological warfare and conducted bacteriological weapon research, but he dodged questions about financial supports, governmental recognition, and other institutes assisting in bacteriological research. Kitano, by contrast, was more cooperative in response to Thompson's investigation.

The following is the record of Ishii's questioning by Thompson:

Q: Who first authorised the beginning of BW research in Japan?
A: There were no orders giving consent to research in BW. If there were, we would have received all the money, personnel, and materials we wanted to carry on this research. Since there were no orders, we only conducted the BW research on a very small scale (1 to 2 per cent) in the Water Purification Bureau.

Q: Who in the War Ministry gave official approval to permit the work to be carried on?

A: The members of the War Ministry did not seem to have any scientific bent. Most of them were of the old school which depended upon the spirit of the Japanese people and not scientific methods to win the war. They did not listen to any of my requests. I did not ask for help directly from the War Ministry. I had to go through channels which meant through the Kwangtung Army.

Q: Did the Kwangtung Army get money from the War Ministry for BW research?

A: I would hand in my requisition for funds. There was no appropriation titled, 'BW'. It all came under Preventive Medicine and Water Purification.

Q: When was the official approval first given to start work on BW and by whom?

A: There was no official sanctioning.

Q: That is hard to believe.

A: If I had labelled my request 'BW' it would have been cut off by the higher-ups. It was all under Preventive Medicine and Water Purification. When I received the money, I used it at my own discretion.

...

Q: Was the commander of the Kwangtung Army in favour of BW research?

A: I never met that man and I do not know what his opinion was.

Q: I cannot see how this work could be done without anybody's approval.

A: I could not achieve what I had planned due to the fact that I did not receive approval.

Q: I am led to understand that you start this work under your own initiative and carried it out on your own responsibility.

A: Yes.

Q: Was the Emperor informed of BW research?

A: Not at all. The Emperor is a lover of humanity and never would have consented to such a thing.[4]

Shirō Ishii concealed many facts from Lt-Col. Thompson; for example, he said he had never met the commander of the Kwantung Army, his direct supervisor, and that 'the Emperor [knew] nothing about the study of bacteriological warfare'. He also stated that 'the Emperor advocates humanism, and he would not agree to such study'. Ishii fully understood that Unit 731 had committed inhumane acts, but he did not halt the study or use of bacteriological weapons, through which he was promoted to higher rank. During his tenure in Unit 731, Ishii was promoted from junior officer to lieutenant-general as an army surgeon. He also ambitiously said: 'Why could not an army surgeon be a captain general? It is unfair!'

Interrogation of Masaji Kitano

Masaji Kitano, the second commander of Unit 731, was interrogated by Lt-Col. Thompson on 5 February 1946. The following is the record of Kitano's questioning by Thompson:

Q: What BW work was conducted at institutions other than at Heibo?

A: Because of the secret nature of BW, no work was done at other institutions.

Q: It is inconceivable that BW research was limited to a single institution, Heibo when other research in Japan, equally as classified, was conducted at many institutions.

A: BW is a restricted subject, prohibited by the Geneva Convention, and thus was not an authorised activity.

Q: Who authorised initiation of BW research?

A: Ishii.[5]

Under interrogation by Thompson, Kitano stated the Unit had done bacteriological warfare research, which violated international treaties and was limited and clearly prohibited by the Geneva Protocol. Kitano made similar statements in his written material submitted to the American military as followed.

I believed that we should have abandoned the research on bacteriological weapons and made efforts to advance the prevention and treatment of communicable diseases. A bacteriological weapon is a misuse of medical science and it was taken up at the Disarmament Conference and the League of Nations as a social problem of international significance. Based upon my own medical knowledge, I think the application of bacteriological weapons for military purposes requires a good deal of work with little to be gained. In fact, we should have no occasion to use it even if we were to complete the study of it, because, for those who are winning a war, it is not necessary to resort to it and thus risk causing an international problem. If those who are losing a war resort to it, the result can only be disgrace. At the beginning of a war when there is no way of telling which side is winning or losing, I firmly believe that the bacteriological weapon is not a decisive weapon.[6]

As commander, Kitano knew that the use of bacteriological weapons was 'inhumane and violation of the international principle' for which he could gain 'notoriety'.

Unit 731 extensively used prisoners of war and civilians as experiment subjects during Kitano's tenure as commander from August 1942 to March 1945, the crucial stage of large-scale production and development of bacteriological weapons. The statements by Shirō Ishii and Masaji Kitano completely contradict their actions. It is obvious that they intended to conceal bacteriological warfare and human experiments, to shirk war crime responsibility, and to evade trial by the International Military Tribunal for the Far East.

The Establishment of Unit 731

To most people in Harbin, China, 5 February 1932 is an unforgettable date: the beginning of humiliation and sorrow. From that day onward, Harbin, a transportation hub of north-east Asia with a population of more than a million, was occupied by Japan as a colony until the surrender of Japan in 1945.

That same year, following his own observation of warfare in Europe, Shirō Ishii urged the use of bacteriological warfare in Japan. After high-ranking soldiers actively persuaded them, many officers of the Imperial Japanese Army General Staff Office and the Army Ministry supported Ishii's suggestion.

Departure from Tokyo: The Beginning of Bacteriological Warfare Research

On 5 July 1932, the Army Ministry approved the establishment of the Bacteriological Research Institute in the School of Army Surgeons, which was later changed to the Research Institute of Epidemic Prevention, of which Shirō Ishii, Ryūji Kajitsuka, Nishimura Eiji, Masataka Kitagawa, Ren Watanabe, Enryō Hōjō, and Hatsutarō Shirakawa were major members. These seven were active members before the foundation of Unit 731 and later became supporters, promoters, and administrators of bacteriological warfare.

Ryūji Kajitsuka later held the office of Secretary of Surgeons of the Kwantung Army; Nishimura Eiji as Head of Unit 1855 in Beijing; Kitagawa as Secretary of the Bacteriological Research, Unit 731; Watanabe as Secretary of 12th Epidemic Prevention and Water Purification Department; Enryō Hōjō (assistant to Shirō Ishii) had worked in the Medical Bureau of the Army Ministry; and Hatsutarō Shirakawa had been the Secretary of 29th Epidemic Prevention and Water Purification in Battlefields.

The aim of the foundation of the Research Institute of Epidemic Prevention is recorded in *50 Years of History of the School of Army Surgeons*:

The Research Institute of Epidemic Prevention as the research institution related to military operations and epidemic prevention in our nation, has recently been founded in the School of Army Surgeons. In 1928, Colonel Shirō Ishii, army surgeon and researcher sent abroad, observed social developments in various European countries, lamented that our nation was not equipped with similar facilities, which was a weakness in national security. After he came back from observations in Europe and the US in 1930, he reported to management about the weakness and suggested that related research should be conducted immediately. Later, Ishii consistently repeated experimental research during his leisure time as a lecturer at the school. With the support of Lecturer Koizumi and approval from the management, a research laboratory headed by Shirō Ishii was set up inside the school.... As the fundamental research of epidemic prevention advanced and in order to practically apply results in battlefields, surgeon Ishii bravely stationed in Manchuria even though difficulties existed, dedicated to the establishment of an epidemic prevention institute. In order to apply the research results and fulfil requests of epidemic prevention from various teams of the imperial military in Manchuria, a new epidemic prevention institute closely attached to the inner inland (the territory of Japan's home islands) was eventually founded in 1936. Certainly, parallel to epidemic prevention research laboratories in the inner island, this institute was the core of epidemic prevention of the imperial military, which was striving for the important mission of epidemic prevention warfare at the stationing area.[7]

On 8 December 1932, the Army Ministry approved a budget of ￥ 208,989 to expand the Research Institute of Epidemic Prevention of the School of Army Surgeons, to increase the number of laboratories, offices, operating rooms, electrical substations, and warehouses, to construct special rooms for breeding small animals, and to produce bacteria of cholera, typhoid fever, and melioidosis. The Institute was able to expand just six months after its founding, reflecting the acceptance of Shirō Ishii and his advocacy of bacteriological warfare by the Japanese military.

As mentioned, 'a new epidemic prevention institute closely attached to the inner inland was eventually founded in 1936'—Ishii's Unit 731. Linked closely to the School of Army Surgeons, Unit 731 became the core of national epidemic prevention; it also assumed the responsibility of 'the important mission of epidemic prevention warfare'. The upper level of the Japanese government also actively drove preparation of bacteriological warfare, which was considered a means of external military invasion.

From Tokyo to Harbin: Establishment of Kamo Unit

After Japan invaded Harbin, its influence spread over the entirety of north-eastern China. In August 1933, Shirō Ishii secretly moved the Research Institute of Epidemic Prevention to Harbin, which is in the Nangang area (Xuanhua Street today). He also secretly set up a laboratory at Beiyinhe, Wuchang city, under the name Kamo Unit, the former body of Unit 731. Ishii also established the Tokyo Branch of Ishii Unit in the School of Army Surgeons where he held office. He commonly travelled between Tokyo and Harbin and conducted research and testing of bacteriological weapons with colleagues, such as Ryoichi Naitō (内藤良一) of the Tokyo branch, in both cities.

Shirō Ishii was born in Chiyoda Village of Sanbu District in Chiba Prefecture, which geographically belonged to 'Kamo Area' at that time; therefore, Unit 731 was named Kamo Unit (see Fig. 1).

Two sections were established under the Kamo Unit: the General Affairs and the Research Section, and under Research were 'Minami subsection' and 'Kotsū subsection'. 'Minami', based at the general office of the Kamo Unit, did research on epidemic prevention and water purification, while 'Kotsū' conducted bacteriological experiments at Beiyinhe, Wuchang city. Beiyinhe was one of the stations along Rafa–Harbin Railway that became a small town after railway construction. As it can be accessed by rail and was near Harbin city, the Kamo Unit built an associated bacteriological factory here, which was disguised as a common barrel of the Japanese military. The Kamo Unit sent a captain named 'Chūma' to manage the facilities at

Beiyinhe, so the site was also called 'city of Chūma'. The city of Chūma was highly secured behind walls more than 3 metres tall, surrounded by moats, sentries at corners, and a high voltage electrical net on the wall.

Beiyinhe Experiment Field: First Base of Human Experimentation

Shirō Ishii had already conducted human experiments at the initial stage of the Kamo Unit. Sanrō Endō visited Beiyinhe on 16 November 1933, writing in his diary:

> ... at 8 a.m., Yasutatsu, Tatsubana and myself visited the Transportation squadron for the development of experiments. The Second Division was conducting poisonous gas and liquid experiments while the First Division was an electrical experiment, and each section applied their experiments on two gangsters. In the gas laboratory, one person was exposed to a poisonous gas, causing pneumonia, which was much worse than yesterday with little life signs today. Another one was injected with 15 ml of potassium cyanate and lost consciousness after 20 minutes. In the electrical experiment, the first person did not die despite repeated electric shocks at 20,000 volts. He was eventually killed by injection. A second person had not died at 5,000 volts. He was killed by burning through electric shock for several minutes.[8]

A year after the establishment of the Beiyinhe Experiment Field, a prison break of 'materials of human experiment' took place on 23 September 1934, the day of the Mid-Autumn Festival, when more than thirty people escaped the prison. Tsuyang Wang, one of the surviving escapees, remembers:

> Half a month ago, Lee and I were walking on a street in Harbin. Suddenly, Kembei (Military Police) and police (City Police) blocked every exit of the street, saying that no matter that they are working, catch them all if they are young and strong. We two were not able to hide ourselves immediately, and we were caught and put onto a truck. More than 40 people were forced onto a train from Xiangfang train station and sent to Beiyinhe overnight. We found something strange after we were jailed. We patiently asked someone who had been sent out and back to the cell, and we were told a secret—that the Japanese used us for bacteriological experiments. Therefore, we decided we could not stay until we died here. We prepared to break jail on the night of Mid-Autumn at the time of meal delivery. On that night, the moon was covered by clouds, and it was raining. Except for soldiers stationed at the watchtowers in the city of Chūma, the rest of the Japanese soldiers were having fun in a restaurant. At midnight, a Japanese guard came toward the cell and delivered a basket of meals and a bottle of wine at the opening of the barriers. I was talking to the drunk guard and picked up the basket, while Lee hit the guard's head when receiving the wine. I then took the key from the guard's waist, he fell down beside the barrier, and I opened the

door of the cell. After that, all prisoners proceeded to the east of the wall under my leadership.

At this moment, the city of Chūma suddenly turned dark because the electricity was shut down, and searchlights were on when we could hear noise from upper levels. Prisoners set up a ladder with their bodies to climb over the wall, and ran east after crossing the moat. Only Lee was left inside as nobody assisted him in climbing the wall. Then understanding what happened, Japanese soldiers started aimlessly shooting and quickly surrounded where we climbed up the wall. Lee was sacrificed with honour.

Chased by soldiers outside the city of Chūma, 20-some of the prisoners were shot and died, while two prisoners were able to escape to Bajiazi, 15 miles away from Chūma. One of them was immediately killed, and the other was transported back to Chūma under escort after they were discovered by Shengsan Wu, a traitor who claimed himself a leader of the self-guarding group. The remaining 12 prisoners escaped to different places: five went to Xinfatun where local people helped them to break their fetters; seven ran to Chengjagang, three miles east of Chūma, to break their fetters and hide there with help from brothers of Zemin Wu and Huamin Wu. At midnight the next day, they joined the team of resistance.[9]

The secret of the city of Chūma was exposed. The first curator of the 731 Museum, Xiao Han, went to Wuchang in 1983 for an investigation of the history in Beiyinhe, collecting oral material from five local witnesses: Zemin Wu, Huamin Wu, Feng Pang, Zhongheng Jin, and Bin Wang. These are now preserved in the Harbin Social Science Academy. In his memoir, recorded on 8 July 1983, Huamin Wu stated:

My home is Chengjiagang, two miles east of the 'Jail of Eastern Manchuria'. On the night of the Mid-Autumn that year, we heard footsteps behind our house. We listened for a short while and heard someone knock and say 'fellows, please open the door'. This was an accent from Shandong. After he opened the door, Wu Zemin, my brother, saw seven people wearing fetters. These seven people said, 'hurry, help us to break these fetters. We escaped from Beiyinhe'.

My brother found an axe and an anvil in the house, calling me to come as well. We led them to a hole of yellow mud. While I kept watching around, my brother broke fetters of several of them but not all. Then I saw flashlights with some noise in the southwest direction. We realised that the Japanese had chased them. We did not have enough time to break all the fetters, and so some of them had broken fetters on one foot. Right after this, we heard the Japanese, and the seven people had run to the east, saying, 'thanks fellows, we will come back in the future'. We went back to the house right before the Japanese entered the village. They did not notice us because we blew out the light. I have not told anybody about this thing, and my brother died after a few years.[10]

Did the Emperor Know?

In order to heighten secrecy and enlarge the bacteriological factory, Shirō Ishii suggested the Imperial Japanese Army General Staff Office transfer the teams related to bacteriological research in 1936. According to 'The Case of Former Japanese Army Preparing and Utilizing Bacteriological Weapons: Judgement Materials', Ryūji Kajitsuka, Secretary of the Kwantung Army, testified when he was standing trial in Khabarovsk:

> Unit 731 was set up based on the order of the Emperor Hirohito in 1936.... The place where the Unit was stationed was confirmed by the headquarters of the Kwantung Army. Before 1941, no official number was assigned for the Unit, and it is usually called the Epidemic Prevention and Water Purification Department of the Kwantung Army as well as the Ishii Unit.[11]

Kawashima Kiyoshi confessed in Khabarovsk:

> Unit 731 was founded based on the secret order of the Emperor Hirohito in 1936, which was originally decided to station in Harbin and headed by the Colonel Shirō Ishii, the army surgeon appointed by the Ministry of the Army. When I took office as the Secretary of General Affairs of Unit 731, I had personally read this order from the archives.[12]

It is widely understood that Emperor Hirohito approved the founding of Unit 731.

In February 2015, we received a copy of a Japanese record mentioning, in a document of the Imperial Japanese Army General Staff Office—'The Document Related to the Approval of Staff of the School of Army Surgeon to Work Part-time as Staff of the Epidemic Prevention Department of the Kwantung Army'—that Prince Kan'in Kotohito (Chief of the Imperial Japanese Army General Staff) gave Terauchi Hisaichi of the Ministry of Army, as well as 'No. 41, Section B of Army Order' in September 1936.

The order stated: 'I ordered to formulate and implement a proposal about staff of the School Army Surgeons working part-time as staff of the Epidemic Prevention Department of the Kwantung Army'.[13] At the end, with approval of the Japanese Emperor, the Chief of Staff, and the Ministry of Army, staff of the School of Army Surgeons could work part-time as staff of the Epidemic Prevention Department of the Kwantung Army. After that, Kotohito issued Terauchi another order: 'This is to inform you that the issue as named in the title was approved by the Emperor as attached. Also, please return the Emperor's approval after reading'.[14] The Epidemic Prevention Department in the document was the name Unit 731 had used.

Under interrogation by Lt-Col. Thompson, Shirō Ishii denied that the Emperor knew of Unit 731. The Emperor not only knew, but also supported the Unit, as shown from the above document, from the personnel size of the Unit at its later stage, from the Unit's budget, and from testimonies of core members.

Barbaric Expansion: Transfer to Pingfang Military Zone

In spring 1936, the Kamo Unit began surveying land in the Pingfang area for a train station site. After the Marco Polo Incident on 7 July 1937, which marked a full-scale invasion of China by Japan, the scale of the Kamo Unit's base had been enlarging as the war went on. Pingfang, a rural village 20 kilometres south-east of Harbin, was also occupied by Japan after Harbin was seized. In 1932, when the Rafa–Harbin Railway was under construction, a station was set up at the south of Pingfang, named Pingfang Station. This village was no different from other Chinese villages in which people had a peaceful lifestyle, but the arrival of the Japanese forced several changes.

Order of the Kwantung Army

The headquarters of the Kwantung Army announced the 1,539th order on 30 June 1938, entitled 'About Setting up a Special Military Zone Near Pingfang'.[15] The zone was secretly called 'the 17th military base'. The order listed several provisions: first, all houses of the Ishii Unit in Pingfang (inside the wall) were designated special military buildings; second, according to 'The Provisions of Implementing Military Affairs Protection Law of Manchukuo', the 'A' lot marked on the attached map was designated a special military zone, in which all prohibitions listed in the above provisions were valid; third, it was prohibited to construct houses of over two stories inside the 'B' lot marked on the attached map; fourth, civil airlines (Manchurian Airline Ltd Co.) had assigned flight routes and no-fly zones; fifth, areas of the 'A' and 'B' lots, as well as all prohibitions, were announced by the Security Department of Manchukuo, while locations of military buildings were announced by the Chief Commander of Defence; and sixth, this order was directly delivered to each related unit, and no circulation of it was allowed.

Afterwards, Harbin City Office set up the Office of Pingfang Special Area Affairs, the Association of Japan-Manchukuo Union in Pingfang Special Area, and Pingfang Police Office. Under the Pingfang Police Office, three local police stations—Pingfang Town Local Police Station, the Third Town of Plain Yellow Banner Local Police Station, and Xinfa Town Local Police Station—were directly administered by the Japanese. Japanese *Kempeitai* in Harbin sent the Pingfang *Kempei* contingent to station Pingfang area, strengthening the uniqueness and concealment of the bacteriological research base.

From a common village to the Pingfang Special Military Zone, this area consisted of Pingfang Town, Unit 8372 of the Imperial Japanese Air Force, the base of Unit 731, and other surrounding areas. This approximately 120-km-square area was divided into 'A' and 'B' zones. Centring at Unit 731 and Unit 8372, a zone was a special control area of approximately 32 km square under strict surveillance of the Japanese military.

Of twenty-five original villages in the 'A' zone, twenty-one located far away from Unit 731 headquarters were preserved, while the remaining four—Huangjiawo Village, Liujiawo Village, Plain Yellow Banner's Fifth Village, and Plain Yellow Banner's First Village—were forcibly destroyed by Unit 731. 'B' zone was a common control area, in which nineteen villages were also under strict surveillance, but comparatively less strictly than those in the 'A' zone (see Fig. 2).

In order to strengthen control over the special zones, the Japanese military installed boundary noticeboards at every transportation hub, 1.5 kilometres away from each village in the zones prohibiting unauthorised entrance. Residents living in Pingfang for generations found the Japanese limited their freedom to enter their homes, and they had very limited freedom of speech (see Fig. 3).

Residents over fourteen years old in the special zones were required to carry a certificate of living, issued by the Police Bureau of Harbin City, and were randomly checked by authorities. Outsiders had to register at the Police Bureau to obtain a temporary certificate of living when they wished to come back and had to cancel their registration when leaving the zones.

One of the certificates issued by Xiangfang Police Station of the Police Bureau is now preserved in the 731 Museum. It was issued to Guo Gao, living at 34, YifaYuan, Xiangfang district of Harbin. On the appendix page, eight items are listed related to entrance restriction:

1. Those living in the special zone over 14 years old must apply for this certificate.
2. This certificate must be carried wherever the holder goes.
3. Borrowing or transferring this certificate is prohibited.
4. Those who move within the special zone must inform police offices at their original places and report to police offices at new destinations within 20 days after arrival.
5. Those who move outside the special zone must apply through police offices at their destinations. After leaving the zone, they must return this certificate to the nearest police office.
6. If any loss or damage of this certificate occurs, holders have to report to and apply for a new one through the police office in charge within 10 days. If the certificate is lost while traveling, holders have to report loss at the nearest police offices and obtain a testimony, and apply for a new one with the testimony after coming back. If anyone finds a lost certificate, he or she must report to the nearest police office immediately.
7. If either the certificate is expired or any information changes, holders must apply for changes through the police office in charge within a month.
8. Violation of the above items would be detained or imposed a fine penalty.[16]

City Within a City: 60 Miles of National Boundary

In 1938, Unit 731 forced a large number of Chinese labourers and drafted many 'special construction workers' from Japan to accelerate the construction of the Pingfang Special Military Zone, where Unit 731 had gradually transferred after construction finished. The original headquarters of the Kamo Unit was preserved as the office of Division Three of Unit 731, also known as the Epidemic Prevention and Water Purification Division. From this time on, the largest scale bacteriological warfare research base in human history was built.

The Unit 731 base and many secret experiment laboratories were located along the Rafa–Harbin Railway connecting Harbin and Chengchun via Xiangfang, Xuanjia, Pingfang, Jioujia, Nyujia, Ralin, Beiyinhe, and Anjia stations. The Japanese military implemented control by setting up secret zones between Xuanjia, Pingfang, and Jioujia stations on the Rafa–Harbin Railway. Every train passing through Pingfang station was required to lower window shades in advance, and passengers were forbidden to look outside. Anyone violating the rules would be arrested by Japanese officials and taken to the Police Bureau or *Kempeitai* under suspicion. The zone seemed to be a city inside a city.

The secret military zone set up along the Rafa–Harbin Railway was commonly called '60 miles of national boundary' (60 Chinese miles, or Li, is equivalent to 30,000 metres). A branch line of the Rafa–Harbin Railway passed through Unit 731's core area of bacteriological research, which exclusively served Unit 731 to transfer 'materials of human experiments' as well as military materials and experimental devices.

Tiny Harbin, Large Pingfang

Facilities of Unit 731 were completed in August 1939, including the general office, Sifanglou (a special prison in the bacteriological research field), experiment facilities, and infrastructure to supply heat, electricity, and water, as well as the exclusive railway and an airport. Additional facilities, such as dormitories, material warehouses, Tōgō Shrine, Tōgō School, Tōgō Square, hospitals, halls, pubs, and sport fields, were also included. The total surface area of Unit 731 core area was approximately 6.1 km square, and a wall 5,000 metres long, 2.5 metres tall, and 1 metre wide surrounded the general office on which high voltage electric webs were installed. Trenches 3 metres wide and deep were dug outside the wall.

Unit 731 resembled a mysterious castle surrounded by military facilities—a high wall, electrical webs, and trenches. Pingfang Special Military Zone was a no-fly zone; even flights of Japanese military were forbidden over the zone, and Unit 731 could shoot them down without advance authorisation. In addition, the Consulate-General of Japan in Harbin and secret connecting points, such as the Jilin Street connecting point, were situated in downtown Harbin outside the head office in Pingfang.

Covertly established by the Japanese Army, and applying biology and medicine in weapon research and manufacturing, Unit 731 conducted inhumane activities in the isolated castle. As Unit 731 became more secretive and its scale grew larger, the rumour of 'tiny Harbin, large Pingfang' spread.

Epidemic Prevention and Water Purification Department

The Ishii Unit formally decreed the use of the name 'Epidemic Prevention and Water Purification Department of the Kwantung Army'. In 1941, the Ishii Unit and other divisions were generally called 'Unit 659 in Manchuria'; the head office in Pingfang, 'Unit 731 in Manchuria'; the Mudanjiang Detachment, 'Unit 643 in Manchuria'; the Sunwu Detachment, 'Unit 673 in Manchuria'; the Linkou Detachment, 'Unit 162 in Manchuria'; the Hailar Detachment, 'Unit 543 in Manchuria'; and the Dalian Research Institute of Health, 'Unit 319 in Manchuria'.

Vast Organisational Structure

The organisation of Unit 731 was huge and consisted of a large number of personnel serving eight departments: General Affairs, Bacteriological Experiments, Bacteriological Research, Epidemic Prevention and Water Purification, Bacteria Production, Training and Education, Equipment Supply, and Therapy.

Apart from these eight departments, there was a special section responsible for prison management. Divisions were set up under each department, sections were created under each division, and each section was named after the person in charge. The General Affairs Department was responsible for writing plans of bacteriological warfare research, drafting unit commands, and personnel, backup, and finance, as well as labour management. The Bacteriological Research Department, as the core institute of bacteriological research in Unit 731, was responsible for researching medicine for offensive bacteriological warfare and producing serum and related defensive equipment. The Bacteriological Experiment Department studied the efficiency of bacteriological weapons and attack methods against humans, animals, and plants. With manufacturing factories for water filters and shells used for bacteriological bombs, the Epidemic Prevention and Water Purification Department was responsible for the epidemic prevention and water purification for Unit 731, and studying and producing bacteriological bombs. Bacteria Production Department developed bacteria, studied and manufactured vaccines, and produced bacteriological weapons. The Training and Education Department trained personnel in bacteriological research, manufacture, and usage, and initiated education of epidemic prevention studies and bacteriological studies. The Equipment Supply Department was responsible for supplying manufacturing equipment, preserving experiment equipment, bacteria, vaccines, and delivering animals for experiment. The Therapy Department provided epidemic preventive methods and medical treatments for members of Unit 731 and their relatives.

On 2 December 1940, Yoshijirō Umezu, commander-in-chief of the Kwantung Army, signed the No. A398 combat command of the Kwantung Army: '… order the Chairperson of the Epidemic Prevention and Water Purification Department of the Kwantung Army to present arrangements of the following units at designated locations: Mudanjiang Detachment—Hailin; Linkou Detachment—Linkou; Sunwu Detachment—Sunwu; Hailar Detachment—Hailar'.[17]

Unit 731 set up the Hailar Detachment, Mudanjiang Detachment, Linkou Detachment, and Sunwu Detachment in accordance with this command. In addition, along with the Dalian Research Institute of Health, which was taken over by Unit in 1938 and transformed as the branch of the Epidemic Prevention and Water Purification Department of the Kwantung Army in Dalian, and a Special Experimental Field and Chengzigou Experimental Field, Unit 731 was comprised of large-scale bacteriological warfare research, production, and testing systems, all provided with vast personnel and comprehensive facilities.

According to the Japanese records of 'Name List of the Epidemic Prevention and Water Purification Department of the Kwantung Army' (関東軍防疫給水部留守名簿), in June 1945, there were four identities, namely general or colonel, officers, soldiers, and dependents. At that time, the Unit had 3,507 members total, including one lieutenant-general, one major-general, seven colonels, four lieutenant-colonels, thirty-five majors, fifty technicians, 135 assistant technicians, thirty-two captains, twenty-three first-lieutenants, twenty-six second-lieutenants, and nineteen chief warrant officers.[18]

Expansion and Spread

The code of the Epidemic Prevention and Water Purification Department of the Kwantung Army was '731'. In reality, this department was one of eight departments of the Kwantung Army responsible for studying water filtration and researching and producing defensive bacteriological warfare equipment. Initiating a large-scale human experiment, Unit 731 prepared and executed bacteriological warfare under the name of 'epidemic prevention and water purification'. Other Epidemic Prevention and Water Purification Departments across Japan and Japan's colonies imitated Unit 731 by claiming themselves 'epidemic prevention and water purification' to prepare and execute bacteriological warfare and human experiments.

According to records from the Ministry of Health, Labour and Welfare, a series of institutions related to bacteriological warfare was founded under direct participation and guidance of Unit 731 from 1938 to 1945. These institutions included Epidemic Prevention and Water Purification Departments of the Northern China Area Army, the Central China Expeditionary Army, the Southern China Area Army, and the Southern Expeditionary Army Group in Beijing, Nanjing, Guangzhou, and Singapore respectively.

Apart from these four, there were still thirty-six Epidemic Prevention and Water Purification Departments of various army divisions, twelve Epidemic Prevention and Water Purification Departments of field operation, and nine independent ones. Until the surrender of Japan, sixty-three units of Epidemic Prevention and Water Purification Departments in total were founded across East and Southeast Asia, such as China, Korea, Malaysia, Singapore, and Thailand.

As Unit 731 was established for invasion and bacteriological warfare, its foundation and development were supported by the Emperor, Japanese Government, the Imperial Japanese Army General Staff Office, the Kwantung Army, and Japan's medical circle. From its foundation, location, scale, and area of Epidemic Prevention and Water Purification Departments, bacteriological warfare gradually became Japan's important means of military dominance of China and other Asian countries. They were crucial components of the plan of invading China, reflecting that Japan's bacteriological warfare was a top-down, premeditated, and organised national crime.

Became Ash: Crazy Actions before Escape

The Second World War reached its final stage in 1945 when most areas of the 'Greater East Asia Co-Prosperity Sphere' came under Allied control. The war in Africa had already ended, Fascist Italy surrendered in 1943, and Nazi Germany unconditionally surrendered on 8 May 1945. Japan was the only remaining Axis power. On 17 July 1945, the US, the UK, and Nationalist China held a conference in Potsdam near Berlin, Germany, and released an ultimatum—the Potsdam Declaration—urging Japan to surrender. On 6 and 9 August, the US military dropped two atomic bombs on Hiroshima and Nagasaki respectively, while Unit 731 in Harbin witnessed some unusual changes.

Destroy Every Evidence: Blast the Headquarters

At midnight on 9 August, Unit 731 received intelligence that the Soviet military launched an attack on the Kwantung Army in the north-eastern China. Shirō Ishii immediately called high ranking military officials for an emergency conference, after which he announced the imposition of a curfew in the station of Unit 731 and prepared for retreat. In order to protect Unit 731's secrecy, Ishii ordered destruction of all command documents, research material, experiment reports, medical equipment, and human specimens.

A surviving labourer of Unit 731, Guozhong Jin, recalls:

> In the night on August 9, 1945, it was raining and planes were flying in the sky. I saw fire on the grassland southwest of Unit 731's station, which was done by Japanese themselves. At 2 am next day, a train arrived on the exclusive track, and those Japanese

independents desperately crowded into the train. After the train left, many Japanese women who were unable to crowd into the train, were crying on the platform. At 3 am or later, there was a very loud sound, and the northwest corner of Sifanglou was exploded by the Japanese themselves. Throughout the day of August, 10 I could hear constant explosions from Sifanglou.[19]

Toshimi Mizobuchi, then Health Corporal of Unit 731, provided the following testimony in 2004:

At around 1 p.m. on August 9, Colonel Kiyoshi Ōta, the Secretary of General Affairs, the Commanding General responsible for blasting the Unit, delivered an order: stop every activity of Unit 731 and terminate Unit 731. Military dependents, according to their level of confidentiality, were protected and transferred back to the mainland by related staffs ... concentrated on the treatment of the 7th and 8th building. On the other hand, a large number of soldiers were working on jobs such as gathering microscopes and burning; remaining military dependents were also doing similar jobs, sending so-called documents, books or X-ray images to the boiler room to burn them.[20]

On 13–14 August, the Ishihara Combat Engineer Battalion of the 131th Independent Mixed Brigade of the Japanese Army bombed major buildings of Unit 731 such as the special prison, Sifanglou, frostbite laboratory, virus laboratory, and tuberculosis laboratory. On 14 August, the last of the Unit 731 staff left Pingfang. Staff from the Mudanjiang Detachment, Linkou Detachment, Sunwu Detachment, Hailar Detachment, and the Dalian Branch also escaped after destroying all evidence.

Massacre of Maruta: Poisonous Air and Hanging

Shirō Ishii ordered Takeo Ishii to deal with the special prison. Takeo Ishii released airborne poison in the prison to kill all *maruta*, and ordered soldiers to shoot *maruta*, even those dead from the poisonous air. Bodies of *maruta* were gathered, doused with gasoline, and burnt for three days.

One veteran of Unit 731 records another bloody scenario in his memoir. *Maruta* were arranged in pairs and given a string and stick. Under surveillance of the special section, standing face to face, each of the pair were looped by a noose around the neck and a stick put inside the noose. One *maruta* held one end of the stick and the other *maruta* held another end, turning the stick in the same direction. As the stick kept turning, the noose became tighter, and the two *maruta* were strangled.

Living under huge pressure, the jailed *maruta* could not easily survive, even if they could escape the experiments. According to investigations thus far, none escaped Unit 731.

Three Prohibitions by Ishii

Standing on the ruins Unit 731's station one rainy evening, Shirō Ishii gave the final order. This was three prohibitions: no one must disclose the identity of Unit 731's members; members must not contact each other; and members must not engage in work similar to that of Unit 731.

Ishii then boarded a flight piloted by his son-in-law, Maj. Miho Masuda, and took some last photographs of the ruins before hurriedly leaving Harbin. Unit 731 completely ceased, and Japan surrendered on 15 August 1945. Members of Unit 731 escaped to Japan via Korea, a few were captured by the Soviet Red Army. These captives stood trial for war crimes in 1949 in the Soviet Union, commonly known as the Khabarovsk War Crime Trials.

Some of Unit 731's members kept the prohibitions and complied with them for a lifetime, which helped cover up the crimes that Unit 731 had committed. Some members violated the prohibitions by engaging in work related to the nature of the unit: for example, Cdr Masaji Kitano, Education Minister, opened hospitals, and Yoshimura, Okamoto, and Tanaka worked in medical schools. Other members maintained close connection after the war and set up many comrade associations, including Pingfang Comrade Association, Tojō Comrade Association, Heihō Sankaku Association, Kamo Association, Gucheng Town Association, and Linglan Association to publicly organise historically commemorative activities. Most of the members, refusing media interviews, have kept Unit 731's wartime secret without discernible introspection.

A very few of them, such as Yoshio Shinozuka, have told the public the truth and bared the historical facts.

Post-War Activities

The Seikonkai, the first comrade association of Unit 731, was founded on 15 August 1955, the tenth anniversary of the surrender of Japan. Its chairperson was Shigeo Suzuki. This was the beginning of large-scale activities held by military surgeons who had avoided prosecution. Later, they built the Seikontō at the Tama Cemetery, Tokyo.

On 15 November 1957, the comrade association published an internal newsletter, *Bōtomo*. Bōtomokai was founded in front of the Seikontō on 17 August 1958, and held its second meeting in Ōtsu City, Shiga Prefecture, on 9 August 1959 and a third meeting on 12 August 1960. In the 1970s, none of the comrade associations were named after Unit 731, and held meetings until 5 September 1981.

Seiichi Morimura described the first meeting of a comrade association in the name of Unit 731. The invitation card read: 'Date and time: 3 p.m., 5 September 1981 (Showa 56) (Sat) (please be punctual); Venue: Satoyamabe Utsukusigahara Hotel, Matsumoto, Shinsyu; Participation fee: 8,000 Japanese Yen. Take a taxi at Matsumoto Station to Satoyamabe Utsukusigahara Hotel'.

Nineteen people from Nagano, Tokyo, Chiba, Kanagawa, and Gunma joined this meeting held in a banquet hall, where a large Japanese national flag was hoisted and a brush calligraphy of 'the first comrade association of Unit 731 in Manchuria, the Kwantung Army' was displayed. At the opening, everyone stood in silence for the war dead, 'for the God of Army, Lt-General Shirō Ishii and officials of Unit 731'.

At the meeting, praise for militarism was highly articulated within a nostalgic atmosphere. One member said: 'It doesn't matter if others know we were members of Unit 731. It is not scary. We were fighting for our nation in those years'. Kawashima Kiyoshi, General Affairs Minister of Unit 731, one of the core members standing trial in Khabarovsk, also sent a congratulatory message. From his message, it is believed that other Unit 731 members might have been invited to the meeting, but they did not attend. Afterwards, one Unit 731 member said: '... nowadays, who will follow Hinomaru and the God of Army? Very few people join this kind of comrade association. We come here not for any war again. Unit 731 is already buried in history, and [we] cannot let the God of Army revive again'.

Shirō Ishii and His Followers

On Wednesday 21 January 2015, Mr Chengmin Jin (金成民) and I were discussing this research project when he showed me a thick old album with the Japanese characters '卒業紀念' (Graduation Yearbook) inscribed in chrysanthemum yellow on the cover. The owner of the album was the president of Kyoto Imperial University and later father-in-law of Shirō Ishii (石井四郎). Although the yearbook dates to 1920, it still looks presentable by today's standard. When I flipped it open, on page two were the stamps of Araki Torasaburō (荒木寅三郎), one written '京大学長' (President of Kyoto University) and the other '天高地厚' (Immense World) in seal characters. The last page listed the publishing committee members. One of them was Shirō Ishii, and this yearbook serves as a key to understand his life (see Fig. 4).

I wonder from time to time whether some people are born murderers, even those who are well-educated. According to the yearbook, Xiaokuan Sun, a Chinese classmate of Ishii, returned to China after graduation. Ishii and Sun, from my point of view, should have shared motives for study at this reputable school. However, their differing experience and destinies made them completely dissimilar. Xiaokuan Sun went on to open hospitals in Shanghai, Guiyang, and other places in China. Dr Shirō Ishii became the prime culprit of biological warfare and human experimentation.

What experience turned Ishii evil? What transformed a well-educated doctor to carry on biological warfare and human experimentation? These inhumane and cruel acts took place in many regions of China during the Japanese invasion in the Second World War—how could Ishii's followers find this acceptable?

Unit 731, biological warfare, and human experimentation are not well-known in the Western world, even though in Asian countries, such as Japan and Korea, the issue has attracted significant public attention.

As a victim of biological warfare and human experimentation, China has been putting effort into encouraging the public to learn the historical facts. In *Deciphering the History of Japanese War Atrocities: The Story of Doctor and General Shiro Ishii* by Kenneth L. Port, the author writes:

Even though Shirō Ishii's activities in World War II cast a long shadow on Dr Mengele's activities in Germany, Ishii is rather quickly being forgotten in the world and especially in Japan. He is no longer taught in high school history or (when he is taught) it is so superficial that few young Japanese people even know the name. In America, no one knows of Shirō Ishii or the carnage he unleashed during World War II.[1]

Compared with national education regarding Auschwitz in Poland, the attack on Pearl Harbor in the US, and the atomic bombing of Hiroshima in Japan, national education about Unit 731 in China still has a long way to go.

Culprits of Biological Warfare: Shirō Ishii

Shirō Ishii was born 25 June 1892 in Chiyoda village, Sanbugun, Chiba prefecture in Japan. Since Chiyoda village is in Kamo area, Unit 731 was also known as the Kamo *Butai* (Kamo Force). The Ishii family is one of Japan's *kazoku* (hereditary peerage) who enjoy the highest privileges bequeathed by the Emperor of the Empire of Japan. Ishii's father, Kei Ishii (石井桂), was a *daimyo* (feudal landholder), someone equivalent to a feudal lord in medieval Europe. Kei Ishii had four sons: his first, Hyōyū Ishii (石井彪雄), died during the Russo-Japanese War (1904–1905), and his second son, Takeo Ishii (石井剛男), was first a peasant in Chiyoda village and then became crematory operator at Unit 731 under the name Takeo Hosoya (細谷剛男) at Beiyin River, Heilongjiang, China. Later, he was head of a special division that managed prisons at Unit 731, and he died on 4 July 1956. The third son, Mitsuo Ishii (石井三男), graduated from a veterinary university in Japan. In 1939, Mitsuo Ishii arrived at Unit 731 where he was the head at the Ishii division that took care of the animal feeding rooms. He passed away on 2 January 1958. The fourth son is Shirō Ishii.

The three brothers were permanent members of Unit 731, and Shirō Ishii used the relationship between family, intermarriage, clan, teacher-student, and classmates to build Unit 731. This recruitment method enabled Unit 731 to continually strengthen its military power, confidentiality, and peculiarity.

Educational Background

Shirō Ishii graduated from Chiba Secondary School and was admitted to Kanazawa's The Fourth High School (金澤第四高等学校) and later Mitoshi High School (水戶高等学校). From 1916 to 1920, he studied medicine at Kyoto Imperial University, which paved a way for his future involvement in Unit 731. He completed three papers in 1920, including 'Study of *Streptococcus pneumoniae*: About bacteriology and biology, Study of *Streptococcus pneumoniae*: About serology, and Study of *Streptococcus pneumoniae*: About toxicity and pathogenicity'. This became his graduation dissertation under the supervision of Professor Kenji Kiyono (清野謙次).

From 20 January to 9 April 1921, Ishii was a probationary officer and lieutenant combat medic in Section Three of Japan's Royal Guards. The following year, on 1 August, he transferred to Tokyo First Military Hospital, where he was promoted to captain combat medic on 20 August 1924. He pursued graduate studies at Kyoto Imperial University from April 1924 to April 1926; thereafter, he continued his job at Kyoto Eijyu Hospital (京都衛戍病院). Under the supervision of Professor Ren Kimura (木村廉), he completed his doctoral degree with a dissertation titled 'Study on Gram Positive *Streptococcus pneumoniae*'. His excellent academic performance impressed the university's president, Araki Torasaburō, whose daughter Ishii married the year he graduated.

Ishii conducted fieldwork observation on biological warfare in Germany, France, and other countries from April 1928 to April 1930. According to the oral narrative recorded by US Army investigator Thompson, '[Shirō Ishii] conducted observations in Egypt, Greece, Turkey, Italy, France, Switzerland, Germany, Australia, Hungry, Czechoslovakia, Belgium, Netherlands, Denmark, Sweden, Norway, Finland, Poland, Soviet Union, United States, Canada and other countries'.[2]

According to Professor Port's investigation, however, Ishii had never been to the United States and Canada. Ishii fabricated this in order to divert the attention of the US Army. The United States Army Forces Command, according to information obtained through a Freedom of Information Act, responded to Ishii's falsehood on 11 July 1991: 'Ishii never visited Fort Detrick or the United States'.[3]

Plague had occurred throughout European history, and the Plague of Justinian (AD 520 to 565) especially interested Ishii: 'Plague continued for 50 to 60 years, spread to almost all notable countries and took the lives of approximately a hundred million citizens'.[4] Regarding the Black Death (1346 to 1665), Ishii noted: '... plague crossed Europe, Asia and the northern shore of Africa, especially the European area. The population of Europe was approximately one hundred million, and one fourth were killed by plague. Half the population of Italy and England died due to the spread of plague'.[5]

From Shirō Ishii's point of view, if *Yersinia pestis* were used as an offensive weapon, it would create massive lethality, which could even wipe out the entire human race. Thus, *Yersinia pestis* was the first choice of biological weaponry for Unit 731. He dreamed to make this insane idea a reality.

Enlistment

Shirō Ishii did not have to wait for too long to see his dream come true. In 1930, he entered the Army Military Hospital as an instructor, a position he held until he passed away. In 1932, while there, Ishii invented a water filter that held a national invention patent and was widely used in the Japanese Army. In 1932, he was promoted to major army surgeon, and on 1 August 1935, he started duty as lieutenant-colonel. Unit 731 was established on 25 June 1936, his forty-fourth birthday.

On 1 March 1938, Ishii was promoted to colonel army surgeon and was awarded imperial recognition of *Shōrokui kunshōdō kūshōkyū* (正六位勳四等功四級) along with core members of the early Unit 731, including Major Army Surgeon Ren Watanabe (渡辺廉) and Captain Army Surgeon Yoshitaka Sasaki (佐佐木義孝), on 5 August 1939.

On 1 March 1941, Ishii was promoted to major general army surgeon, and on 1 August 1942, he was sent to Northern China to be first captain army surgeon, with the assistance of Masaji Kitano (北野政次) as vice-captain army surgeon. Ishii retuned to Unit 731 on 1 March 1945 and was promoted to lieutenant-general army surgeon.

Three days before Emperor Hirohito announced Japan's surrender, Ishii sneaked back to Japan from Harbin on 12 August 1945 and a year later was investigated by Arvo T. Thompson, Norbery H. Fell, Murray Sanders, and other US military officers. By providing the US Army with abundant documents and data regarding biological warfare and human experimentation, these Japanese war criminals escaped their war crimes trials.

Doctor Who Met Shirō Ishii: Michinobu Haga

The fifteen-member Japan Christian Medical Association visited our International Research Center of Unit 731 on 8 June 2015. The Center held a small-scale seminar for the group. One member, Dr Michinobu Haga, born in Changchun, China, in 1933, worked at the *Kokuritsu* Tokyo *Daiichi Byōin* (First National Hospital of Tokyo) in 1959, where he first met Shirō Ishii.

At the seminar, Haga revealed:

> I met Shirō Ishii at the hospital [First National Hospital of Tokyo] during autumn. Shirō Ishii stayed at the single ward. He was seriously ill. The nurses and everyone who came to visit him called him Ishii *Kakka* [Your Excellency]. We had a brief conversation. I told Ishii that I was born in Manchuria and stayed there for a while before I returned to Japan. Shirō Ishii replied to me that 'it should be a tough experience' and so on. It was like a day-to-day conversation.

Before Shirō Ishii died, people around him were still calling him *Kakka*, something considered unusual today.

Haga met Ishii the autumn before Ishii died of throat cancer. Fukiko Aoki (青木富貴子) wrote in her book *731*: 'Shirō Ishii was a pedantic, posturing and talkative officer who was able to fool the Military Headquarters of Japan. Because of surgery, however, he lost his voice, and died soon. What a mockery for him!'[6] Shirō Ishii had funeral services at both the Buddhist temple Gekkeiji (月桂寺) in Tokyo and his hometown Kamo. Ishii's successor, Masaji Kitano, organised the memorial services.

The Successor: Professor, Doctor and Lieutenant General Masaji Kitano

Biography of Masaji Kitano

Masaji Kitano was born in Hyogo prefecture, Japan, on 14 July 1894. He graduated from the School of Medicine at Tokyo Imperial University on 26 November 1920 and became a second-class army surgeon on 7 March 1921. From 1 April 1923 to 1 March 1925, he studied infectious disease, especially intestinal perforation and shigella, at the graduate school of Tokyo Imperial University.

On 13 November 1923, Kitano was promoted to first-class army surgeon. On 1 April 1925, Kitano withdrew from graduate school and obtained his doctoral degree in medicine from Tokyo Imperial University, where his dissertation was titled 'Experimental research on seronegative intestine perforation and paratyphoid fever'. On 1 August 1929, he was promoted to *Santō guni sei* (chief third-class army surgeon).

In August 1932, Kitano served at the First Army School and held a teaching position at the Medical Department of the Ministry of War of Japan. From 12 January to 11 September 1933, he made visits to Europe and the United States for research. He received a medal from the Emperor of Manchukuo for his contribution to its establishment. He was then promoted to *Nitō guni sei* (chief second-class army surgeon) on 1 August 1935. The following year, Kitano worked at the headquarters of the Kanto Army as a professor of microbiology at Manchukuo Medical University (see Fig. 5).

Army Surgeon to University Professor: Tokyo to Changchun

Before moving to Changchun to become professor of microbiology at the Manchukuo Medical University, Masaji Kitano was an army surgeon. To transfer his profession from that to professor in Manchukuo was a complicated process. The CEO of South Manchuria Railways Co., Yōsuke Matsuoka (松岡洋右), submitted a report, 'About application for recruitment of full-time professor', to the Minister of the Army Terauchi Hisaichi (寺内 寿一) on 30 June 1936. The report stated: '*Nitō guni sei* Masaji Kitano is suitable for the post of professor at Manchukuo Medical University. Therefore, according to the following requirements, now we hire him at the University to be a full-time professor'.

As Kitano was a *Nitō guni sei* at the time, Matsuoka offered him ￥ 3,000 per year as salary, with an allowance and bonus worth 40 per cent and 45 per cent of the salary, and housing allowance that was less than 40 per cent of the salary for his duty as professor in Manchukuo Medical University, which made his total yearly salary around 6,750 YEN. According to *Bukka no sesō 100nen* (*100 Years of the Situation of Commodity Prices*) by Jirō Iwazaki (岩崎爾郎), the price of rice was ￥ 0.24 per kilogram in 1935.[7] In other words, Kitano's annual salary could purchase 281,215 kilograms of rice, enough for a family of four for thirty-eight years.

On 20 August, Minister of the Army Terauchi Hisaichi submitted the application to Prime Minister Hirota Kōki. The next day, it was approved and Kitano succeeded to the position at Manchukuo Medical University.

Research Papers of Masaji Kitano

The Japanese Association of Medicinal Sciences held an academic conference for bacteriologists featuring group photographs taken in front of the famous Yasuda Auditorium at the Tokyo Imperial University. In this photograph, Shirō Ishii is fifth from left in the front row, fourth from right in the same row is Masaji Kitano. It is the only photo of the two that we have found. In contrast with the scientists, they are in military uniform and hold sabres. It is uncertain whether Ishii and Kitano participated in the conference as doctors, scholars, professors, military, or other roles (see Fig. 6).

As shown below, we have found that Kitano wrote more than thirty research papers between 1931 and 1939 in *Gunidan zasshi* (Army Surgeon Magazine) that appeared during wartime. From the contents and number of papers, Kitano was a scholar who made contributions to the field. It is clear that both Kitano and Ishii shared a number of similarities: they were both doctors of medicine, professional researchers, lieutenant-general army surgeons, commanders, and pioneers in carrying out bacteriological warfare and human experimentation (see Fig. 7).

Chart 1: Research papers published by Masaji Kitano in *Gunidan zasshi*

Number	Title	Year and volume
1	'Based on the Start of Hiroshima Army Preparation Hospital'	1931 Vol. 204
2	'About the Process of Smallpox Vaccination'	1931 Vol. 205
3	'Observation of the Statistics on Dengue Fever among Japanese Army'	1931 Vol. 220
4	'Three types of Statistics on Dysentery among Japanese Army '	1931 Vol. 221
5	'About Bacteria Carrier Symptoms among Imperial Army'	1931 Vol. 223
6	'About Description on Freeze-Dried Smallpox Vaccine'	1932 Vol. 223
7	'Investigation on Infectious Disease'	1932 Vol. 225
8	'About Statistics on Early Precaution of Infectious Disease Carriers'	1932 Vol. 230
9	'About Statistics on Early Precaution of Infectious Disease Carriers'	1932 Vol. 231
10	'Research on Enteric Fevers and Paratyphoid among Japanese Army (First Report)'	1932 Vol. 232
11	'About Reaction after Vaccines for Enteric Fevers and A Type and B Type Paratyphoid'	1932 Vol. 232
12	'About the Type of Dysentery among Japanese Army'	1932 Vol. 233
13	'Observation of the Statistics on Food Poisoning among Japanese Army'	1932 Vol. 233

14	'Observation of the Statistics on Carries of Enteric Fevers and Paratyphoid after Vaccine'	1932 Vol. 234
15	'About the Reaction of Vaccine of Plague'	1933 Vol. 234
16	'About the Result on Dysentery Vaccine and Medicine among Japanese Army'	1933 Vol. 234
17	'About Regulations of the Conference on International Armed Force Medical'	1933 Vol. 246
18	'About International Regulations of Medical Plane'	1933 Vol. 246
19	'About the Function and Duty of Committee of International Armed Force Medical Conference'	1934 Vol. 247
20	'About the Latest Trend of Medical Plane'	1934 Vol. 248
21	'About Automatic Washing and Disinfection Machine'	1935 Vol. 267
22	'About Prevention of the Spread of *Encephalitis lethargica* in Japan'	1935 Vol. 269
23	'About Dysentery Carriers among Japanese Army'	1935 Vol. 270
24	'About Research on the Popularity of Dysentery among Japanese Army (First Report)'	1936 Vol. 282
25	'About *Ophthalmic Myiasis* in Mongolia'	1937 Vol. 299
26	'About Air Transportation of Injured Red Army'	1937 Vol. 301

Masaji Kitano was released from Shanghai on 9 January 1946. Upon his return to Japan, he was investigated by the US Army on 6 February. He submitted a seventeen-page written statement regarding Ishii's troops on 1 April 1947. Early in the war, Masaji Kitano was also a member of the Japanese Expedition First Antarctica Special Committee and Pertussis Research Center, set up by the Ministry of Education, Science and Culture.

After the death of Shirō Ishii in October 1953, Kitano became the person in charge of Ishii's funeral. In 1971, Japanese reporter Katsuichi Honda visited the former Manchukuo Medical University at Shenyang, where he discovered the statistics on human experimentation that appeared in many of Kitano's research papers. When Honda returned to Japan, he interviewed Masaji Kitano by telephone, but Kitano either kept silent, refused to reply, or rejected Honda's narrative. In the 1970s, Japanese television broadcasting company TBS attempted to interview Masaji Kitano, who refused the interview request, saying, 'I want to forget what happened in Unit 731. I do not want to recall that memory.' The TBS reporter continued: 'Do you mean human experimentation?' Kitano replied, 'Yes.' Public materials pertaining to Masaji Kitano remain undisclosed since then. On 17 May 1986, Kitano died at the age of ninety-one.

Hisato Yoshimura: Principal of Kyoto Prefectural Medical University and Head of Frostbite Laboratory at Unit 731

Biography of Hisato Yoshimura

Hisato Yoshimura (吉村寿人) was born in 1907 in Hyogo prefecture, Japan. He studied at the School of Medicine in the Kyoto Imperial University from 1926 to 1930 and was elected student union chairperson. After graduating, Yoshimura was hired by Professor Rinnosuke Shōji from the School of Medicine as his assistant in the Department of Physiology for the research project 'PH measurement of blood'. In 1936, Yoshimura received a doctoral degree that allowed him to start his career as lecturer in physiology. On the recommendation of Professor Rinnosuke Shōji in 1938, he joined Unit 731 as a technician in the first frostbite experiment laboratory.

Yoshimura returned to Japan from Harbin in August 1945. In September, he became a lecturer in the Aeromedical Studies at Kyoto Imperial University. Nine months later, in 1946, Yoshimura worked as a professor of physiology in Hyogo Medical University (now the Department of Medicine of Kobe University). The principal of the university was Yoshimura's former teacher, Professor Rinnosuke Shōji. Yoshimura transferred to the Department of Physiology in Kyoto Medical University and started long-term research, including a paper titled 'Physical Effects of the Lack of Protein'. In 1962, Yoshimura was elected chairperson of the Japan Weather Association, and was president of Kyoto Medical University from March 1967 to 1969. He left the University in March 1970. Before he took over the post of professor in Hyogo Medical University, Yoshimura was a professor at Kobe Women's University, head of the Pollution Research Center in *Kyusei Kaikan*, and held other positions. In 1978, Yoshimura was awarded the Order of the Rising Sun Third Class. Two years later, he retired from his position in Hyogo Medicine University and transferred to Kobe Women's University again. He died 29 November 1990 at the age of eighty-three.

Human Experimentation by Hisato Yoshimura

Hisato Yoshimura conducted frostbite experiments in Unit 731 from 1938 to 1945 as a member of the human experimentation team. He was the first in medical history to use living human beings for such experiments. The archaeological site of Unit 731 preserved the large-scale frostbite experiment laboratory. Yoshimura and his team members chose to conceal the truth, and none of them provided accurate oral accounts of the events. The author can only rely on Yoshimura's research papers and other oral accounts from old veterans in understanding what took place in that laboratory.

Oral Accounts of Frostbite Experiments on Living Human Beings
Nishi Toshihide, a former chief of the training and education division of Unit 731, stated during the Khabarovsk war crime trials:

I read the report written by Hisato Yoshimura about human experimentation. Regarding this point, there was a video. The video showed four to five people in fetters put outdoors. They were wearing cotton garment and had bare hands. Later, a huge electric fan was put in front of them to speed up the process of frostbite. Then their hands were hit by a small wooden stick to check if they were already frostbitten.[8]

Military police of Unit 731 Kurahara explained:

When I walked into the laboratory at the prison, I saw five Chinese men sitting on a bench. Two of them had already lost all their fingers. Their palms were dark. Bone was visible on the hands of the remaining three Chinese men. Although they still had their fingers, they were just finger bones.[9]

Frostbite Experiment on a Hundred People

After the end of the Second World War, Yoshimura published an article titled 'Research on Skin Reaction under Severe Cold' in *Physiology Society of Japan*. Yoshimura used 100 Chinese civilian men and women, aged from fifteen to seventy-four, to observe the reaction of humans in water of 0 degrees Celsius. Judging by the number of civilians used in a single experiment, one can conclude that Unit 731 had an abundance of test subjects, and using subjects of different ages could provide relatively comparable data.

Human Experimentation on a Baby

According to the same research paper, 'Research on Skin Reaction under Severe Cold', Yoshimura conducted experimentation on a three-day-old baby. He put the baby's fingers into 0-degree Celsius water for thirty minutes daily for a month.

To a normal human being, such action is unimaginable. There is no way to conduct it without help from a third party, and what kind of human could witness such cruelty to a baby and jot notes? We were particularly interested in understanding their thoughts at that time. Who was the baby? Where were the parents? These questions remain unanswered, and the life of the baby is reflected only in statistics in Yoshimura's paper.

Yoshimura lived to the age of eighty-four. As a father and grandfather, what were his thoughts about his own children? Did he ever think of his past when he was with his family? Where was his conscience with that baby? He was educated in an upper-class institution, but where had his human nature gone?

Results of Human Experimentation Applied in War

For eight years, Hisato Yoshimura's frostbite division conducted human experimentation on human beings of varied nationality, age, and gender. His work was supported and praised by the Japanese Kwantung Army as well as the Ministry of War of Japan. The experiments and research were filmed as promotional documentaries, and the data were used as educational materials for the Japanese Army to avoid frostbite in wars against China and Russia.

Life after the Second World War and Academic Results

Under the protection of the US, Hisato Yoshimura escaped the International Military Tribunal for the Far East. His acts in Unit 731 were forgotten by the public. The experimental data and statistics gained from his dirty and bloody acts in Unit 731 were permanent contributions to Japanese medical development. Yoshimura was appointed principal of the Kyoto Imperial Medical University, chairperson of the Japan Weather Association, and held other important roles in universities and research centres. In addition to research papers, he published several books, including *PH Theory and Measurement*; *Kwashiorkor: The Theory and Fact of Protein Nutrition*; *Medical Psychology: Adaptability of Humans—Case Study on Adaption to Climate Change*; *Summary of Human Physiology*; *Outline of Medical Psychology*; and more.

Memoir of Hisato Yoshimura

On Hisato Yoshimura's seventy-seventh birthday, he wrote *Kijyu kaiko* (*Memoir of My 77th Birthday*). In this book, he said: 'I published my research outcomes during wartime in the English Physiology Magazine and received massive feedback from Western scholars. Even now, these are major references not only in Japan but many universities and research centers in the world'.[10]

From this statement, Yoshimura seems to be a leader in the field, but where did his statistics come from? All these useful materials were from his abundant cruel human experiments. Those such as Yoshimura, who committed medical crimes and war crimes, should have been tried and imprisoned for what they did in Unit 731 instead of spending their rest of lives publishing and giving talks on their 'data'. Yoshimura, however, did not regret his acts in Unit 731. When he was interviewed by reporter Tomizo Asano (朝野富三) from *Mainichi Shimbun*, Yoshimura claimed: 'It was war. All the evil is due to the country, and is the country's responsibility'.

A Kyoto physician, Dr Ichiro Kadowaki (門脇一郎), published an article titled 'Former Principal of Kyoto Imperial University Hisato Yoshimura and Unit 731' in which he wrote:

> They called the people who conducted human experimentation and their forced guinea pigs as 'contributors' to the improvement in medical progress and research on frostbite prevention and recovery from frostbite for the Japanese Army. This is discrimination on human beings. From the principles of health and value of life, it was an unfair and selfish statement toward all mankind. The inventors took away the property of victims, not only material life, health and property, and even their basic human rights. Did they have the right to do so? This is a fundamental mistake. Everyone is equal. Everyone has the right to life and health. The fundamental purpose of medical development is to support and uphold basic rights for all mankind. It is not allowed to break this rule for

any reason. And it is not possible to give up the right of anyone for other's happiness. Of course, to give up other's right, no one can gain happiness.[11]

Errors in the Hundred-Year History of the School of Medicine at Kyoto University

Reflections of Two Memoirs

I visited the School of Medicine at Kyoto University in 2010. When I was talking with Professor Nagahiro Minato (湊長博), director of the school, he explained that there was another Minato, Masao Minato (湊正雄). He and this Minato had no connection.

Professor Minato gave me a book with a long and interesting title in both English and Japanese, *Curiosity, Challenge and Continuation: Kyoto Daigaku Yigakubu Shoritsu 100 Shuunen Kinen Arubamu* (*Curiosity, Challenge and Continuation: The Centennial Memorial Album of the School of Medicine of Kyoto University*), published in 2004. Back in Harbin, I briefly flipped through the volume and placed it on the shelf as one of many reference books never to be read again. Later, I had a chance to read the Graduation Year Book of 1920 from the same medical school in Kyoto. When I placed the two books side by side and compared the photos and records in both, I was surprised to have found Shirō Ishii missing.

The two books shared some similarities: the same people appeared in both, including the president of Kyoto Imperial University Araki Torasaburō and the professors from the School of Medicine, such as Ren Kimura, Kenji Kiyono, Seiwa Tanabem, and Shosan Toda. These men were Shirō Ishii's teachers and had inseparable relationships with Unit 731.

The 2014 book is divided into pre-war and post-war sections. Shirō Ishii is nowhere in the album, only his teachers. As a graduate of bachelor, master's, and doctoral classes in the School of Medicinem, as well as a lieutenant-general, Ishii merits inclusion in the memoir greater than that of his teachers. What is the reason for omitting him from the university history? Famous Japanese writer Seiichi Morimura once wrote: '… the truth should be kept and history cannot be left empty'. What is the rationale for not including Ishii in the *Centennial Memorial Album*? It is clear that the School of Medicine of Kyoto University deliberately omitted those graduates who served in Unit 731. Will this act make the school history more perfect?

Records in the Shirankai Name List

I received the document *Shirankai Name List* by chance; its former owner was Kai-ji Yang (楊開濟), a 1941 graduate of the School of Medicine of Kyoto University. His personal information is recorded in the list: 'Kai-ji Yang, Republic of China, internal medicine, lives in Republic of China Beijing Xicheng District Shoubi Hutong No. 13'. The list was published on 20 December 1942. The editor and publisher was Toshio Nishimura (西村敏雄) and the list was published by the Shirankai Corporation of Kyoto University's Medical School, founded 1906, which served the alumni of the School of Medicine.

By 1942, there were forty sub-branches of alumni associations, including thirty-four in Japan, such as Tokyo sub-branch and Kyoto sub-branch, sub-branches in various parts of China, including Taiwan, Dalian, Fengtian (Shengyang), Harbin, and Jiamusi, and a Gyeongseong (renamed Seoul in 1945) sub-branch in Korea. The Harbin sub-branch was once located in the Medical University in Harbin. Ikuharu Narita (成田幾治), who wrote the first book on medicine in Harbin, *Medical History of Harbin*, was in charge of the Harbin sub-branch.

The sub-branch in Harbin consisted of twenty-four persons in 1942: Susumu IKawakami (川上漸), Kinzo Takadome (中留金藏), Tarō Sonoda (園田太郎), Hisato Yoshimura, Tachiomaru Ishikawa (石川太刀雄丸), Kōzō Okamoto (岡本耕造), Seiwa Tabe (田部井和), Masao Minato (湊正男), Hideo Tanaka (田中英雄), and Hiroyuki Suzuki (鈴木啟之) were permanent members in Unit 731.

According to Shirankai records, members were graduates, current students, graduate students, professors, associate professors, lecturers, assistants, and staff of the School of Medicine of Kyoto University. Other than that, professionals from a medical field could apply for membership in Shirankai with permission of board members. From the record, PhD students such as Shirō Ishii and Keiichi Noguchi (野口圭一) from the School of Medicine of Kyoto University joined Unit 731 with honours as graduates of a top ranked university.

Members of Unit 731 on the Shirankai Name List in 1942					
Number	Name	Subject	Degree	Graduate Year	Post
1	Susumu Inoue (川上漸)	Pathology	Doctor	1909	The First Pathology Division in Unit 731
2	Shirō Ishii (石井四郎)	Micro-organism	Doctor	1920	Vice-division head
3	Masasuke Tamada (玉田政助)	Internal Medicine	Doctor	1925	Army Medical College, Army Surgeon Lieutenant-Colonel
4	Kinzo Takadome (中留金藏)	Pathology	Doctor	1926	Army Surgeon Colonel
5	Yukisada Masuda (増田之貞)	Micro-organism	Doctor	1926	Army Medical College, Army Surgeon Colonel

6	Tarō Maruta (園田太郎)	Pathology	Doctor	1928	Army Surgeon Lieutenant-Colonel
7	Yoshitaka Sasaki (佐佐木義孝)	External Medicine	Doctor	1930	Army Surgeon Lieutenant-Commander
8	Hiroyuki Suzuki (鈴木啟之)	---	Doctor	1930	Army Surgeon Colonel
9	Hisato Yoshimura (吉村寿人)	Biology	Doctor	1930	Army Technician
10	Tachiomaru Ishikawa (石川太刀雄丸)	Pathology	Doctor	1931	Army Technician
11	Kōzō Okamoto (岡本耕造)	Pathology	Doctor	1931	Army Technician
12	Seiwa Tabe (田部井和)	Micro-organism	Doctor	1931	Assistant Professor, Department of Medicine
13	Ryoichi Naitō (內藤良一)	Micro-organism	Doctor	1931	Army Medical College, Army Surgeon Lieutenant-Commander
14	Masayoshi Hirasawa (平澤正欣)	External Medicine	Bachelor	1933	Army Surgeon Colonel (Public)
15	Masao Minato (湊正男)	Micro-organism	Doctor	1935	Army Technician
16	Susumu Shibata (柴田進)	Internal Medicine	Bachelor	1937	Army Surgeon Lieutenant-Colonel (Public)
17	Kōzō Okamura (丘村弘造)	Medical	Bachelor	1937	Army Surgeon Lieutenant-Colonel (Public)
18	Akira Itō (伊東詮)	---	Bachelor	1937	Army Surgeon Lieutenant-Colonel
19	Junichi Kawamura (河村純一)	Internal Medicine	Bachelor	1937	Army Surgeon Lieutenant-Colonel
20	Keiichi Noguchi (野口圭一)	---	Bachelor	1937	Army Surgeon Lieutenant-Colonel (Public)

21	Hideo Tanaka (田中英雄)	Dissection	Doctor	---	Division Head, The Fourth Bugs Division

Those on this list were Ishii's teachers, fellows, and comrades-in-arms. To pursue their experience on the battlefield and in post-war times is a challenging task, since written documents about them remain undiscovered.

Green Cross Japan and Unit 731

In November 1950, Ryoichi Naitō and Hideo Futaki (二木秀雄), the head of the Tuberculosis Division of Unit 731, co-established the 'Blood Bank Joint Stock Company' to produce blood products in Japan. Ryoichi Naitō was manager of the Epidemic Prevention Research Center, which Shirō Ishii had held as a colonel. Naitō was also manager of the Ishii Troop headquarters in Tokyo. He gained respect and trust from Shirō Ishii and later played an important role in dealing with the US after the end of the Second World War.

The company was renamed 'Green Cross Joint Stock Company' in 1964. Masaji Kitano joined the company as a director and president of the Tokyo sub-branch. Kurobuta Ichirō Ota (大田黒猪一郎) from the Epidemic Prevention of Southern Army became the president in the Kyoto sub-branch. More than ten members of Green Cross were former members of Unit 731.

At the outbreak of Korean War, Ryoichi Naitō used his special relationship with the US to supply the US Army with dried plasma and earn a fortune. In the 1980s, the news of blood products infected with AIDs shocked the country, and the Green Cross was one of the defendants in the case.

Doctor Susumu Kawakami: Teacher and Subordinate of Shirō Ishii

Susumu Kawakami graduated from the School of Medicine of Kyoto Imperial University and was Shirō Ishii's pathology instructor. Kawakami was also a major member in the Harbin sub-branch of Shirankai. From 1937 to 1942, he worked in the Pathology Division of Unit 731, and simultaneously taught at Keio University as a professor of pathology.

In February 2015, I read some twenty handwritten drafts by Susumu IKawakami in the Unit 731 archive. Kawakami had written these letters to friends—including Yu Akimoto and Kenji Kiyono of Unit 731—and they were written in Japanese using Chinese brushes; his handwriting looks nice from the perspective of Chinese calligraphy.

An excerpt from Kawakami's letter to Yu Akimoto on 20 November 1942 shows in detail his work life—with significant omissions:

I have been in Harbin for five years. This year is the fifth winter. This January I moved to a place near the headquarters. Since the heating system is good in the dorm, I did not feel cold even though it is minus twelve to thirteen degrees. The workshop headquarters temperature is about 23 degrees, and I need to remove my coat. Depending on conditions, [I will] slightly open the window to let fresh air in. When the external air meets internal air in the room, it becomes mist, so it is hard to see each other one inch away.

The workload is not busy, but it is not possible to relax. When work becomes busy, especially under emergency conditions, [I need to] work intensely. If not, [I can be] more relaxed. [I come to] Manchuria in such an intense period, no matter what, I work until today, and I live my days without worry and fear. I wake up at 5 am, usually read scripture five times, [drink] one cup of *matcha* [a type of green tea], and after one cup of *sencha* [a type of green tea] I recite Avatamsaka Sutra for about 500 words. I eat breakfast at 8 am, start working at 9 am and am off at 5pm, take dinner at 6 pm, shower at 8 pm and go to bed at 9 pm. This is my daily life. I live on the third floor in a single room.[12]

Among these letters, as from the medical divisions of Unit 731, there is no mention of war or medical research.

Even though they were strictly monitored by the Unit, it would have been impossible not to mention the nature of their work. From our point of view, they were not allowed to lie, but they did not dare tell the truth to their family and friends. In this way, they were a group of lonely and evil medical experts working in a division that killed hundreds while they themselves were living in peace. Is that the reason for his Avatamsaka Sutra-reciting habit, in order to wash away his guilt and for salvation?

One of Kawakami's handwritten letters mentioned two letters written to him by Isoroku Yamamoto (山本五十六), the officer later charged with orchestrating the attack on Pearl Harbor. It is strange that the two made contact. In 1944, when Kawakami died in Tokyo, his funeral was arranged by Shirō Ishii, which also indicates a close relationship between Kawakami and Ishii.

Veterans Tell the Truth

On a rainy night in August 1945, before the escape of Unit 731 staff, Shirō Ishii ordered all members to keep the records top secret—a secret that should go to their graves. Ishii himself, however, failed to do so. Facing the prospect of trial by the US Army in Tokyo, he revealed the truth about Unit 731 along with abundant documents in return for his escape from trial.

Ishii's daughter, Harumi Ishii (石井春海), told *The Times* on 29 August 1982: 'As far as I know, it was true that a deal was made. But it was the US side which approached my father, not the other way around.... What I would like to emphatically say ... is:

Isn't it important that not a single man under my father's command was ever tried as a war criminal?'[13]

There are many who hold the same view as Harumi Ishii. In fact, most members of Unit 731 believed Shirō Ishii saved their lives. Ishii's daughter, his subordinates, and even Ishii himself ignored the most important issue: they covered up the inhumane nature and unethical war crimes conducted by Unit 731. Members of Unit 731 spent the remainder of their lives in a peaceful, dignified way and indeed brought the story to their graves.

Some members, including Yoshio Shinozuka (篠塚良雄), Fukumatsu Okawa (大川福松), Toshimi Mizobuchi (溝渕俊美), and Sadao Koshi (越定男), did not go with the majority and revealed the story to the public.

Yoshio Shinozuka

Yoshio Shinozuka was the member of Unit 731 who revealed the truth in the most honest and active way. He was only fifteen when he joined the Unit in 1939, and until he went back to Japan, when he was thirty-two years old, Shinozuka spent seventeen years in war. He said: 'I was like a stranger at that time'. Yoshio Shinozuka , formerly named Yoshio Tamura (田村良雄), was from Chiba prefecture like Shirō Ishii. When Unit 731 collapsed in 1945, he joined the Liberation Army led by the Chinese Communist Party. In 1952, Shinozuka turned himself in to the Liberation Army, confessing he was a former member of Unit 731 and was later confined in the Fushun War Criminals Management Centre.

In 1956, the Standing Committee of the National People's Congress promulgated 'About the decision for the management of war criminals of Japanese invasion of China'. The Supreme People's Court of the People's Republic of China announced the release of 1,017 Japanese war criminals who had been charged with lesser war crimes and had exhibited good behaviour. Yoshio Shinozuka was one of these and was set free on 28 July 1956. A number of those released from Fushun War Criminals Management Centre established the Association of Returnees from China (中国帰還者連絡会) whose purpose is to reveal war crimes by the Japanese Army in China and to encourage friendship between China and Japan. Shinozuka is a permanent member of the Association. He was often at the peace gatherings held in Tokyo and Hiroshima in Japan, as well as in Harbin and Changde in China.

On 25 June 1998, Shinozuka was invited by the San Francisco-based Global Alliance for Preserving the History of World War II in Asia (世界抗日战争史实维护联合会), of which the co-author of this book, Professor Yue-him Tam, was the Executive Vice-President, to give talks in the US and Canada. However, Shinozuka was denied entry at the Chicago international airport and repatriated back to Japan because he was identified as a war criminal on the confidential list newly established by the Department of Justice in the United States, for the following reason: '… participated in inhumane behaviour during WWII'.

After fifty years, ironically, the country that once exempted members of Unit 731 from trial showed concern for human rights. The US seemed to forget how it exempted Unit 731 from guilt. Those veterans who spoke the truth, and those who did not, are free to enter the US, and even Ryoichi Naitō, the key figure in the trade between the US and Japan during the trials, is able to visit the US. Why were those brave enough to face and speak the truth in public, such as Yoshio Shinozuka , rejected by the US? Is this because Shinozuka spoke out before the entire world instead of exclusively and privately to the US?

In 2005, Shinozuka, then age eighty-three, visited the site of Unit 731 where he demonstrated the use of the bacteria incubator. The following year, he participated in the Second International Conference on War Crimes in Biological Warfare held at Chengde, China. As a former member of Unit 731, Shinozuka had connections with many Chinese historians and family members of victims.

As time goes by, there are fewer eyewitnesses from Unit 731 willing to tell the truth. On 20 April 2014, Shinozuka, aged ninety-two, the last veteran of Unit 731 willing to talk about the past, passed away at his home in Chiba, Japan.

Fukumatsu Okawa

In 2008, the Heilongjiang Broadcasting Television decided to produce the documentary *Immortal Memory*, commissioning Mr Chengmin Jin and his crews to Japan to visit Fukumatsu Okawa (see Fig. 9).

Fukumatsu Okawa, formerly named Fukumatsu Murada, was born on 18 August 1920. He worked at the Beian Army Hospital and later transferred to Unit 731, where he participated in 'live human body dissections'. Due to his hard work, Okawa gained praise from Shirō Ishii and was awarded a military sword. Following his interview with the television crew, Okawa offered to donate the sword to Harbin, and wrote the donation letter to the Harbin Government. Unfortunately, the donation to Harbin failed, but his handwritten narrative reveals a gruesome truth:

I joined the Medical Division of Japanese Army in Showa 15 (1940). Later I was appointed a job in the Beian Army Hospital. After three months of training, I started working at the pathology laboratory immediately. We used mice, guinea pigs, apes and other kinds of animals for experiments of typhoid fever, dysentery, plague and cholera to observe their reaction. At the same time, we did regular check-ups for the soldiers on their sputum, stool and pee. For the controversial issue 'comfort women' [sexually enslaved civilian women and girls], there were 30 to 50 of them in different divisions, and we did regular check-ups on syphilis for those women. The Beian Army Hospital was also responsible for daily experiments on human bodies and animals under the command of Shirō Ishii. To use gluten to produce penicillin was the reason to join Unit 731 in 1944. At that time, I knew I entered no ordinary place. Why did I reach this conclusion? Because there were three rules for us to obey: 'do not see, do not speak and do not listen'. Under these three rules, I had to do research on different viruses, rickettsia and other things every day. Especially on frostbite, cholera and plague experiments on human and used human bodies to make specimens. Those human beings used in experiments were called '*maruta*'. They had no names, just numbers. There were Russian, Chinese, Korean and Japanese. These were people under criminal punishment. All their names were undisclosed and were secrets, too. I did not feel good at the beginning. I could not work well. After several days, I was getting used to it. I did dissection on two to three, five at the most, human bodies each day. I observed the condition of the frostbite, syphilis, plague and cholera-infected humans, and put the viruses into glass bottles. At the same time, I needed to work with several people from the Yoshida Division for blood cultivation and conducted enrichment medium with egg incubators. My former name was Murada Fukumatsu. I changed and hid my identity when I returned to Japan.[14]

Toshimi Mizobuchi

A Japanese gentleman, Masataka Mori (森正孝), donated some of his video interview footage of veterans of Unit 731 to the Unit 731 International Research Center. Among these videos, the interview with Toshimi Mizobuchi in September 2004 is extremely valuable.

Toshimi Mizobuchi joined the Hayashiguchi Division of Unit 731 on 1 April 1943. In March 1945, he was transferred to the headquarters of Unit 731. Before the retreat of Unit 731 after the end of the Second World War, he was appointed to head the 'Unit 731 Destruction Division'. When Masataka Mori asked him the purpose of the establishment of Unit 731, Mizobuchi replied:

> I think the purpose of Unit 731 was to attack by using bacteria and to protect us from similar attacks by our enemies. Because biological and chemical warfare were banned under the International Convention, many countries in the world were secretly doing certain research. The existence of Unit 731 has been the biggest secret of our country [Japan]. From my point of view, our Unit was established under the protection of the entire country [Japan].[15]

Toshimi Mizobuchi commented on Shirō Ishii's merits: 'Ishii had three doctoral degrees: medicine, pathology and engineering. His research dissections on the Ishii-style water filters allowed him to obtain doctoral degrees in pathology and engineering. The foresighted-Ishii introduced preventive healthcare to the army'.

Mizobuchi's narrative confirms the motive and method of destruction of Unit 731: on 9 August, Unit 731 established 'Unit 731 Destruction Headquarters'. General Division Head Sumimasa Ota (太田澄) was appointed Head Commander. The Division started destroying the special prison block 7 and block 8, killed the imprisoned 'testers', and burned all the research documents and experimental equipment.

On 9, 10, 11, and 12 August, around 2,000 members of Unit 731 were divided into three batches and took the dedicated railway to leave the *pingfang*. The train passed through Changchun, Siping, Tonghua, Pyongyang, Gyeongseong, Yongsan, and finally arrived in Busan. In the afternoon of 24 August, Shirō Ishii arrived in Busan. The members of Unit 731 eventually went back to Japan from Sengi, Hagi, Susa, Hakata, and other places.

On 12 August, Unit 731 worked with Ishihara sappers to put bombs around the site and bombed the Sifanglou; on 13 August, they bombed the boiler room of Dynamics Division; and on 14 August, at 2 p.m., Shirō Ishii flew back to the headquarters in Harbin by plane. He made an order—'the train will arrive in two hours. All staff in the headquarters must get on the train and leave'.

According to the oral narrative of Toshimi Mizobuchi: 'Unit 731 continued putting fuel on each building and set them afire. Once it was on fire, there would be surprisingly massive sounds of explosion. When people saw from the train, without any order (to do so), they saluted the burning site. I think it was similar to when ancient people saw the fall of a castle town'.

Sadao Koshi

Sadao Koshi, from the Transportation Division of Unit 731, was a driver for Shirō Ishii. He also transported 'humans' a few times. 'Human' in this context here means 'human beings for experimentation'.

In 1994, Koshi accepted an interview request from scholar Masataka Mori:

... although this is banned by the International Regulation, things happened two months before the defeat [of Japan] were too impressive to me. Me and Sergeant Nakayama were on the way to collect *marutas*, about 40 pieces, which means 40 people, all white Russian. Every time [we transported them] to the fixed destination, which was Sifanglou. [We] translated to the *marutas*: 'now we are going to give you vaccination. Come down one by one.' Then we killed all 40 people one by one by potassium cyanide. Why did we kill them all? Because there were too many experimentees, and we could not send them back to the consulate. Since they were useless, we killed them all.[16]

Koshi continued:

At Anda testing ground, [we] tied the legs and hands of the 'experimentees' on the cross, placed an iron-made plate on their chest, and these 40 people were placed in a circle. Inside the circle, we put about 25 grams of bombs. The bombs sometimes carried virus for plague, sometime cholera or anthrax. Observers retreated 4,000 meters away from the circle. They set a timer for the bombing and observed the 'experimentees' being infected.[17]

In the book written by Sadao Koshi, he wrote:

In February 1944, at Anda testing ground, one experimentee escaped before the bombing. When me and Nakayama noticed, he was out from the cross. He started to help the others to get out from the cross. When we went towards the crowd, all 40 people escaped and ran away in all different directions. Because they all had fetters on their legs, they were not able to run far. We used our car to hit them one by one. Human lives are so fragile. Just one hit and they are gone.[18]

In 1983, Sadao Koshi published *Hinomaru ha akai namida ni* (*Bloody Tears on Hinomaru*) exposing the events at Anda testing ground of Unit 731.

In 1994, Koshi revealed in an interview:

I am so tired now. After the book was published, I was blamed by multiple telephone calls, and more than 1,000 letters were sent to my home. [The threat was like] 'Why do you reveal the truth? I will kill your family.' At 2 and 3 a.m., I was blamed every moment. I was really about to go crazy. I put a cotton blanket on the telephone and put it inside the closet eventually. I almost did not get out of the door. Because of the book, I was completely turned into a victim.[19]

From this oral narrative, we understand most of the veterans who chose to reveal the truth were lower ranking employees of Unit 731. Due to their status in the Unit, they were not able to get to the core secrets of the Unit. Their exposed information can hardly be compared with the rich information of Unit 731 given to the US by high-ranking core members who supplied the US with important data and statistics as well as experiment reports.

Core members in the Unit supposedly sworn to keep secrecy, did not keep secrets for the country. When their lives were threatened by trial, they chose to abandon the *Bushidō* spirit and pride of militarism in exchange for their pardon. After the investigation by the US, these members never spoke again about the truth publicly. Even so, could they really spend the rest of their life in peace?

Leading by the Elites: Crimes by Doctors of Medicine

It is clear that, as represented by Unit 731, Japanese Army Hospitals, Field Hospitals, and the Epidemic Prevention and Water Purification Departments committed various organised medical crimes, such as bacterial warfare, human experimentation, frostbite experiments, and live body dissection. As these war crimes have been covered up and denied in the mainstream in Japanese society, they therefore have remained unresolved, creating challenging issues and strained relationships between China and Japan.

Most army surgeons in Unit 731 were alumni of famous Japanese universities. They were elites who held doctoral degrees in bacteriology, serology, epidemiology, cryptozoology, entomology, and botany. First division head Shirō Ishii graduated from the Department of Medicine Kyoto Imperial University, and second division head Masaji Kitano, as well as being the head of general division Kawashima Kiyoshi (川島清), held doctoral degrees from Tokyo Imperial University. These elite men became core members of the management and decision makers for the initiation of human experimentation and biological warfare.

As medical experts and elites, doctors should serve their country with conscience, observe international medical regulations and medical ethics, and bear responsibility to help the needy. In the grip of extreme militarism, these men abandoned their consciences and carried out human experimentation and biological warfare. They chose to become war criminals and committed crimes without considering their role as doctors or their medical ethics. Their cases reflect how Japanese citizens and society ignored international regulations and social order under the influence of extreme militarism.

After the Second World War, these medical doctors escaped the Khabarovsk War Crime Trials. They should have been imprisoned, but they rose to socially prominent positions in Japanese Government and military departments. The leader of the Anthrax Division, Hajime Uemura (植村肇), became the chief textbook investigator of the Ministry of Education, Science and Culture; Minao Nagatomo (長友浪男) became the vice-governor of Hokkaido; Junnichi Kaneko (金子順一) became the chief investigator of Ministry of Defense; Hideyoshi Nakakuro (中黒秀外之), the principal of Health School in Ministry of Defence; and Miho Masuda (増田美保), professor in the National Defence Academy of Japan. Those who were in medical services, including the head of Plant Research Division Yukimasa Yagisawa (八木澤行正) and the head of Dysentery Research Division Shinpei Ejima (江島真平), joined staff at the National Institute of Infectious Diseases. Shiro Kasahara (笠原四郎) from Virus Research Division was appointed as the vice-director of The Kitasato Institution.

Some former members of Unit 731 started careers in academic institutions and universities. Hisato Yoshimura from the Frostbite Division was appointed principal of Kyoto Imperial University, while the head of Pathology Division Tachiomaru Ishikawa became principal of Kanazawa University. Kōzō Okamoto, the former member of Pathology Division, worked at Kyoto University as chairperson in the Department of Medicine. Head of Entomology Hideo Tanaka worked at the Department of Medicine in Osaka City University. The head of Typhoid Fever Division Seiwa Tanabe and the head of Cholera Division Masao Minato were appointed professors in Kyoto University. Tadashi Miyagawa (宮川正) from the X-ray Division became a professor in Tokyo University. Several members of Unit 731, such as Toyokichi Eguchi

(江口豊潔) from The Third Division, Tarō Sonoda (園田太郎) of the Education Division, and Keiichi Noguchi of the Plague Division, established their own medical enterprises and private hospitals. They enjoyed lives of wealth and security.

Those who escaped trial became key members in post-war Japan and sowed the seed of the resurrection of militarism. Indeed, the lack of proper prosecution of war crimes has had serious effects on post-war Japanese society. Just as there was no proper trial for many war criminals such as members of Unit 731, Japan's Emperor Hirohito remained innocent of his responsibility in the aggressive war against China. All these unsolved issues paved the way for the rise of the far right-wing in Japan, and the amendment of history textbooks resurrects Japanese militarism in modern Japanese society.

After the War, Stories from Victims' Families

'Special transfer' or 特移扱 (*tokuitatsukai* in Japanese) was a unique term used by the *Kempeitai*, Police Unit, Security Unit, and Special Agencies of Unit 731. It originated with human experimentation in Unit 731: the Japanese captors referred to those who were specially transferred as 'luggage' and '*maruta*'. These people suffered capture, torture, and imprisonment, and finally died due to experimentation, vivisection, bacterial infection, and other cruelties.

Introduction to Special Transfer

What is Special Transfer?

Takeo Tachibana, one-time head of the *Kempeitai* in Jiamusi, said:

> ... when I was the leader in the Jiamusi *Kempeitai*, we often chose prisoners from the *Kempeitai* to Unit 731 for experiments. We followed the order of the *Kempeitai* headquarters and pre-trialled them. We did not refer their cases to court but sent them directly to Unit 731. This was a special method, which was called the special transfer.[1]

Former Kanto *Kempeitai* vice team leader Torao Yoshifusa explained in Fushun War Criminals Management Centre:

> Since the Mukden Incident, Japanese imperialism allowed Japanese soldiers to kill Chinese civilians who provoked protests among Chinese society. The Japanese imperialists had to change their strategy toward the Chinese. On the surface, they announced the abolition of serious punishment of Chinese civilians, but later on, a secret agreement was reached among Kanto *Kempeitai* Commander Ueda Kenkichi, Staff Hideki Tojo, Army Surgeon Shirō Ishii, Staff Nagaoka

Machitake, Kanto *Kempeitai* Commander Tanaka Shizuichi, Chief of Police Unit Kajisako Jiro and Officer Matsuura Kokki that arrested Chinese civilians who fought the Japanese Army should be sent to the Ishii division for human experimentation use.[2]

Victims sent by special transfer included Chinese, Russians, and Koreans. They were prisoners of war from the Chinese Kuomintang (Nationalist Party), the Chinese Communist Party, guerrillas, and the Russian Red Army, Chinese and Korean intelligence operatives hired by Russia, and civilians including peasants, workers, and merchants.

Undifferentiated Ultimatum: Standard of Special Transfer

The Kanto *Kempeitai* and its sub-groups were major participants in special transfer. On 26 January 1938, the Kanto *Kempeitai* headquarters published a command document about special transfer, and on 12 March 1943, the headquarters further announced 'Ultimatum of Special Transfer', which set comprehensive regulations about special transfer.

The new regulations stated 'those criminals who will be released or soon be released after brief confinement by the court', 'those committing no serious crimes but not recommended to be released', 'people who have no fixed residence and relatives', and 'opium addicted individuals' should be sent to Unit 731. The new standard for special transfer was so broad that it failed to restrict the power of the *Kempeitai*, which subsequently could arrest and kill Chinese criminals and civilians indifferently, and could decide who should be a special transfer for Unit 731.

Special transfer as recorded in the collected documents went through the following process. First, Unit 731, in order to conduct human experimentations, needed a large number of 'testers'. The Unit communicated that number to the headquarters of the *Kempeitai* in the Guandong region (Northeastern China), the *Kempeitai* and its sub-groups arrested civilians in secret for the Harbin *Kempeitai*, and victims were specially transferred to Unit 731 in Harbin. To receive a large number of 'testers', the Unit set up a *Kempei* office that initiated contact with Harbin *Kempeitai*.

Sadao Koshi, Ishii's driver at Unit 731, wrote in his book *Hinomaru ha akai namida* (*Bloody Tears on Hinomaru*) about four locations to receive 'testers': the *Kempei* office near Harbin train station, the intelligence agency in Harbin, the headquarters of Harbin *Kempeitai*, and the Japanese Consulate in Harbin.[3] Victims were kept in the special prison and could be released as 'living testers' for human experimentations at any time. It is particularly shocking that the Harbin Consulate, the highest diplomatic authority representing Japan, acted as a secret connecting point and hub for 'testers' exchange, equipped with an underground prison that kept '*maruta*' for Unit 731.

Revealing the Truth about Special Transfer

Two important publications have exposed the details of the special transfer. The first one is in Russian entitled *yianskayia Krasnayia Armiyia. Primorskiĭ voennyĭ okrug. Voennyĭ* tribunal (*Trial Materials of Preparation and Use of Bacterial Weapons by Former Japanese Army*), published by Moscow Foreign Languages Publishing Raboche-Krest in 1950; the second book is in Chinese, *Xijunzhan yu Duqizhan* (*Bacterial War and Poison Gas War*), published by the State Archives Administration in China in 1989. The two publications recorded oral narratives about special transfers from eyewitnesses Yutaka Mio, Torao Yoshifusa, and Tetsuichi Kamitsubo.

That the Japanese army carried out special transfer was confirmed in the 1950s, but there was no official written record of it until October 1997, when Chengmin Jin discovered a document in the Heilongjiang Province Archives. Scholars began to search out families of the victims named in those records.

The families of victims of special transfers are a large group of individuals. When I contacted them, I found that most of them are living in ordinary lives but suffer deeply in their hearts. They searched for their family members but failed numerous times. Some of them only saw pictures of their fathers, and some remembered only a vague image of their fathers. A number of them died without knowing where their fathers went or whether they were alive. People who live in the post-war era may not remember the disaster brought by the Second World War. For families of victims, war brought perpetual nightmare and pain (see Fig. 8).

When History Encounters Reality: Victims Meet Perpetrators

In the afternoon of 10 April 2015, my colleagues, Ms Rujia Liu and Ms Tongzhu Wang, and I took a train to Shenyang to meet with Yibing Wang, a member of victim Yaoxuan Wang's family. Since summer 2005, the year when I first met with Yibing Wang, I have met with him at least once a year for academic activities and media interviews. Although I met with Wang more than ten times, I never met him in his hometown Shenyang. I especially wanted to understand his life there.

In the morning of 11 April, we visited the Palace of the Qing Dynasty, a UNESCO World Heritage Site. Light rain started to fall that afternoon, and I was standing by a window looking at the busy street. I was thinking how tiny humans are when compared with the big city, when Xiaoguang Wang—Yibing Wang's son—knocked on the door. We rode to Wang's home at 11 Wanrong Road.

He and his wife were home in their tidy two-room flat of about 60 square metres and welcomed us with oranges and apples. Yibing Wang was born in 1930. His hearing and vision were both good, but his response was a bit slow. Yibing Wang has four children and one grandson from each child (because of China's one-child policy, most families have one child). Yibing Wang was thirteen years old when Yaoxuan Wang visited him at Beijing Huiwen Primary School. It was the last time he saw his father.

Yaoxuan Wang, born in 1898, was originally from Zhanglukou village at Raoyang, Hebei. He joined the Chinese Communist Party in 1939 and served as correspondent and Soviet spy. He lived at 24 Xinglong Street, Beijing City, and was the owner of *Hongtaihao*. In 1941, he opened Xingya Photo Gallery and Fuxing Stationary at Dalian. The two shops were the International Far East information exchange station with Delong Shen as manager and led by Zhongshan Li and Baozhen Wu, who were spying on the Japanese Army. In the autumn of 1943, Manchuria Unit 86 discovered secret radio waves in Dalian that sent signals to Chita, the Soviet Union, and Yanan, China, every Tuesday and Friday at midnight. They tracked the radio waves to Fuxian Stationary at 153 Shijiaosha, Dalian. At midnight on 1 October 1943, eighty soldiers from the Dalian *Kempeitai* took over Fuxian Stationary and arrested Delong Shen, Guiqin Liu , Wenhua Li, and Yaqin Li. The *Kempeitai* searched the shop and found the radio, wires, code book, and other evidence.

According to investigation records of the Japanese Army, Delong Shen, born in 1911, was from Raohe of Dongan at Manchukuo, joined the Northeast Anti-Japanese United Army in 1934, and later studied at the Communist University of the Toilers of the East. He was fluent in Chinese, Russian, and Korean. Shen later joined the Soviet Communist Party. In December 1939, sent by the Soviet Red Army, Shen became a radio waves intelligencer. During trial by the Dalian *Kempeitai*, Shen revealed information about the organisation, members, activities, communication codes, and passwords of the International Far East Information Station.

Xingya Photo Gallery was closed by the Dalian *Kempeitai*, and Zhongshan Li and Baozhen Wu from Fuxian Stationary left that day for Shenyang to pass the news to Shenyang Information Station. The Dalian *Kempeitai* collected information from Shen in a short period and, according to Shen's information, started large-scale arrests.

On 6 October 1943, the Dalian *Kempeitai* arrested Zhongshan Li, Ziguang Han, and Jiechen Shi in Shenyang. On 11 October, Yaoxuan Wang and his niece, Xuenian Wang , were also arrested by the Japanese *Kempeitai*. *Kempei* Yutaka Mio and Setsu Naganuma extorted confessions by torturing, beating their legs with wooden sticks, feeding them chili water, putting them on an electric chair, and striking them with a soldering iron.

Subsequently, Dalian sent Yaoxuan Wang, Xuenian Wang , Zhongshan Li, and Delong Shen to Unit 731 by special transfer arranged by Yutaka Mio, with the approval of *Kempeitai*, under the charge of being 'Soviet intelligence officers'. The rest of the arrested Chinese disappeared after the accusation. That was the mystery of the influential Incident of Dalian Heishijiao (see Fig. 10).

The disappearance of Yaoxuan Wang has worried Yibing Wang and his family all these years. After the surrender of Japan in 1945 and the establishment of People's Republic of China in 1949, there was no news of Yaoxuan Wang. In 1955, the Martyr Certificate of Yaoxuan Wang was sent to Yibing Wang confirming his father was killed by the Japanese. Yibing Wang has suffered greatly from the loss of his father, and for fifty years after his father was killed, he attempted to collect materials about his fate.

Beginning in the spring of 1993, he searched the archives in Beijing, Shenyang, Dalian, Changchun, and Harbin for anything regarding Yaoxuan Wang.

In 1994, Yibing Wang engaged attorneys Hiroshi Oyama, Toshitaka Onodera, Harumi Watanabe, and Shogo Watanabe to bring a suit against the Japanese Government. In preparing material for the suit, Harumi Watanabe found Yutaka Mio, the former member of Dalian *Kempeitai*. Watanabe explained to Mio about Wang, including his desire for an apology from the government to the family, assumption of complete responsibility for the loss of Yaoxuan Wang, and asked Mio to be witness in the law suit.

Yibing Wang recorded the response from Harumi Watanabe when he explained the situation:

> Harumi Watanabe said the person who '... arrested, tried and special transferred your father and your cousin to Unit 731 was Yutaka Mio'. I was shocked at that time. It seemed like all the sorrow and anger became clearer. I did not want to listen anymore, but I could not help wanting to listen to the lawyer's explanation of how he found Mio.

Harumi Watanabe told Yibing Wang:

> Yutaka Mio was specially amnestied to Japan in 1956. He regretted his behaviour that gave pain and suffering to the Chinese, and he decided to prevent the rebirth of Japanese imperialism. In order to improve the relationship between Japan and China, and to maintain world peace, he and other amnestied Japanese soldiers established the Association of Returnees from China with Mio as one of the committee members. After his return, he worked hard for improving Sino-Japanese relationships and therefore he received pressure from the right wing in Japan. Mio could not find a job and suffered a hard life. But he continues working hard to reveal the war crimes committed by Imperial Japan.

Yibing Wang, his cousin, and his younger sister listened and did not speak a word. Harumi Watanabe continued: 'On January 5, 1994, when Yutaka Mio and Setsuji Nagane travelled to China, they visited the Dalian city government and made their apologies to the Chinese for their special transfer of Yaoxuan Wang to Unit 731 when both of them were members of Dalian *Kempeitai*'.

Yibing Wang watched Watanabe stop in the middle of the conversation. 'And I tried hard not to cry in front of a Japanese,' he said (see Fig. 11).

On the fiftieth anniversary of the victory of the Sino-Japanese War in 1995, the Anti-invasion and Peace Maintenance Seminar was held in Harbin. Both Yibing Wang and Yutaka Mio joined the seminar. On 31 July, accompanied by Yuan Jin, former manager of the Fushun War Criminals Management Centre, Mio apologised to Yibing Wang. The following is the narrative from Yibing Wang about his meeting with Yutaka Mio:

At 7.30, I, Xiaoguang Wang, Wenjun Shi and Ying Liu from the Dalian Chronicle Office gathered in a small conference room at the Harbin Airport Hotel. Wenjun Shi and Ying Liu provided me information about Dalian *Kempeitai* in the past. When we were seated, Yuan Jin came over, and an extremely thin and humpbacked individual followed him. His eyes were hollow, and his hair was all grey. He seemed to be in his 80s. He was Yutaka Mio.

Yuan Jin came two steps forward. Since he was tall and big, he stood between me and Yutaka Mio to prevent contact between abuser and victim. He spoke in fluent Japanese: 'this is the family member of martyr Yaoxuan Wang, Yibing Wang'.

Later, he pointed to the thin old man and spoke to him in Chinese, 'This is the former member of Dalian *Kempeitai*, war criminal Yutaka Mio, the abuser of martyrs Yaoxuan Wang and Dongsheng Wang'.

During the introduction, Yutaka Mio bowed deeply and didn't move a bit. When Yuan Jin finished the introduction, he moved forward and kept bowing, at the same time, kept saying: 'I am guilty, I am guilty…'

Yuan Jin repeated in Chinese. It began the conversation between us with Japanese and Chinese translation by Yuan Jin.

'Dear family member of martyr Yaoxuan Wang, Yibing Wang, I am guilty. I followed the imperialist aggressors of Imperial Japanese to China and started a mad invasion'.

Wenjun Shi and Ying Liu took out their cameras and two precious pictures. I listened to Mio's apology and felt increasingly angry. Had I not been a Communist Party member, I would stand up and beat him up. My discipline and rational power helped controlling my anger.

'When I was Sergeant Major in Dalian *Kempentai*, I arrested your father and cousin at Tianjin. Because of my guilt, I bought serious disaster to the two families. I am guilty. I apologise to your family. The policy of "hate the crime but not the individual" from the Chinese government made me a new person, saved me and gave me a second chance to live. This allowed me to make apology to you. Not only did I torture your father, more seriously I sent him to Unit 731. They died in there [Unit 731]. It was all my fault. My guilt was as serious as leader of bacterial warfare Shirō Ishii. Once again, I apologise to you all, and all family members of the victims. I will regret for my entire life and fight for the friendship between China and Japan. I am willing to reveal the truth done by imperial Japan during WWII and become the witness for Mr [Yibing] Wang. Once again, know I will apologise to all members of Chinese victims, especially to both of your families, forever'.

After the conversation, Yutaka Mio bowed deeply again (see Fig. 12).

I listened to the apology from the abuser of my family and myself, and I thought of my relatives who participated in anti-Japanese activities and suffered under pressure and died. I kept calm and restrained my emotions. I coughed and spoke slowly, 'you arrested my father and cousin, tortured them and sent them to

Unit 731. They died from human experimentation. Your guilt is serious. There is hatred between us. Your guilt is inevitable. It will be recorded in the history of imperialist aggressive actions by Imperial Japanese Army. With the surrender of Japan, you were kept in the Fushun War Criminals Management Centre and you deserved this. Within more than 10 years of that sentence, you admitted your aggressive action and regretted your crime. You were specially amnestied by the Chinese government. Now you transformed from a war criminal to a new person, and regained the right to become a new man. And you came back to China and apologised to the Dalian city government. Today you apologised to the victims, which means you accept your new life. In Chinese society, we have a saying "it is never too late to mend". Now you accepted the fact of your war crime, and it is forgivable. But you have to keep your word and become a person who is beneficial to Sino-Japanese friendship. Do not be duplicitous.'

Yutaka Mio listened to my words. He kept his head down, wept and bowed. The meeting lasted for more than ten minutes.

In 1995, Yibing Wang sued the Japanese Government in Tokyo for the first time. On 16 August, Yutaka Mio apologised to Yibing Wang again. This time Yutaka Mio knelt in front of Yibing Wang, and Wang finally shook hands with Mio. Within one month, Mio had apologised to Yibing Wang twice—in Tokyo and Harbin. There was a sentence on a Japanese review of the event saying 'handshake over hatred', and I wondered about the hatred between Yibing Wang and Yutaka Mio. What did they feel? How can one handshake compensate for national disaster?

On 22 September 1999, the Tokyo District Court announced the result of the Unit 731 case:

… the court decided that during 15 years of war against the Chinese, the aggressive action of the Japanese army was against humanity and the fact of aggressive action was proved by a variety of evidence and materials. The oral narratives given by victims and witnesses were true and reliable. The Japanese government should sincerely apologise to the Chinese civilians. Relationship between Japan and China is basic to the two nations. No matter happened in the past or will happen in the future, in order to maintain the friendship between the two countries, the Japanese government must understand its importance.[4]

Lastly, Judge Go Ito said: '… personal suffering due to war should be settled at the national level, and a government has no right to give response'. Yibing Wang's appeal was ultimately rejected.

After the rejection, Yibing Wang was depressed. He visited the Unit 731 Museum and took some soil from the ruins. He bought the soil back to Shenyang in a bag, put it into a cremation box, and considers it his father's ashes. The box is in the cemetery of martyrs in Shenyang today.

On 29 July 2004, Yibing Wang sued the Japanese Government in Tokyo once again and failed. In 2005, the case was sent to the Supreme Court of Japan. The Court rejected Wang's appeal by reason of 'the right to claims against Japan has been given up by the Japan-China Joint Communiqué'. From 1995 to 2013, Yibing Wang went to Japan five times, but any apology and reparation from the Japanese Government are yet to come.

I asked Yibing Wang, 'When would you think of your father?' Wang thought for a while, no one made a sound in the room among the five or six people present. He finally said, 'After my father was arrested by the Japanese, all these years, I missed my father. After the surrender of Japan, I missed him even more. Why didn't he come back?' Yibing Wang sighed and continued, 'I have lived to this age, and my children and grandsons are grown up, I don't want to think of it, don't want to think of anything.' I saw him use his shaking left hand to wipe away tears, then he was silent.

I asked Yibing Wang, 'How is your life now?' Yibing Wang said, 'I am quite good. Now I am retired from a copper wire factory at Shenyang, and my salary increased a while ago. Each month I receive a pension of more than 2,400 Chinese *yuan*. I had a hematencephalon and myocardial infarction and stayed at the hospital for a while. Now I am fine.'

When the meeting was about to end, Yibing Wang signed his name on my notebook and we took a few photos together (see Fig. 13).

As I was about to say goodbye, I felt very sad. The rain had stopped and the sky was misty. On the way home, although I was with my colleagues, I felt lonely. We boarded the train to the next station, Changchun, where we would meet with Fengqin Li, the next family member of a victim of a special transfer.

Victim of the Second World War in a Peaceful Period: Fengqin Li

On 12 April 2015, we took the train D8095 from Shenyang to Changchun. There were few people in the compartment, and despite the sound of the train, the atmosphere was quiet. I have visited Changchun numerous times, and as an historian, I often think of its history before arriving there.

Eighty years ago, Changchun—renamed Shinkyo by the Japanese—was the capital of the puppet state Manchukuo, and Aisin Gioro Henry Puyi ruled as puppet emperor of Manchukuo for twelve years. The city, once the centre of power of Imperial Japan, is the provincial capital of Jilin, and it is well-known internationally as the home of First Auto Works (FAW) Group Corporation. Among its many well-preserved historic buildings, the most famous is the 'Manchukuo old eight part' including the Military Department (Sheriff's Department), Ministry of Justice, Ministry of Economic Affairs, Ministry of Transportation, Ministry of Agriculture, Ministry of Education, Department of State and Department of Livelihood.

At 6.30 p.m., bilingual announcements reminded us to disembark the train. We arrived at the new Changchun West Station.

On the morning of 13 April, three of us visited the Museum of the Imperial Palace of the Manchu State, and that afternoon, we went to the home of Fengqin Li.

I have known Fengqin Li since 2009. In November, she and I visited Japan and submitted the 'application of family members of victims of special transfer' to the Japan Parliamentarians' Union, expressing anger over human experimentation during the Second World War.

As a scholar and a victim, we also supported the suit against the Japanese Government by the victims of biochemical warfare. I had previously introduced Li to a reporter from *Harbin Daily* for an interview, and she appeared on the news a few times. Today, as a researcher, I felt different seeing her again (see Fig. 14).

Li lives on the first floor of a three-bedroom apartment of about 100 square metres, usually with her son. At her home, Li made dumplings and prepared fruit for us. After lunch, she told me she has two sons and two daughters, and each of them have one child. The family are living a relatively comfortable life. Then we talked about Li's father, Pengge Li (see Fig. 15).

My father Pengge Li, also named Fuchang Li, was born on July 12, 1917 in Xiongyuecheng sutun, Geping of Liaoning Province [now Liming Village at Xiongyue, Yingkou city]. He graduated from the Department of Communications in Fengtian Railway Campus. Li married Guilan Su in 1937, and one year later my brother Zhigui Li was born. Li worked at Mudanjiang railway station and lived in the dormitory at the Jinling Street, Mudanjiang. In the summer of 1941, my father was arrested by the Mudanjiang *Kempeitai* and sent to Harbin *Kempeitai*, and later died in Unit 731 at the age of 25. I was born half-a-year later and I never met my father. [See Fig. 16.]

In 1958, my brother Zhigui Li applied to the Chinese Communist Party and needed to undergo a family background investigation. Someone claimed that my father died of an unknown cause, so my brother did not get into the Party. In 1975, Zhigui Li applied to the Party again, Yingkou city again checked his family background. Investigators found that Pengge Li had worked at Mudanjiang railway station and concluded that 'Pengge Li was a good man'. So, Zhigui Li finally joined the Chinese Communist Party. Because of his application, I knew there was someone who knew about my father's past in the Mudanjiang railway station, and therefore I started to check my brother's application materials.

The application included a detailed narrative of Naijia Zhou, a colleague of Pengge Li, written on 1 September 1975:

I graduated from the Fengtian Railway Campus in spring 1938. I worked at the Hengdaohezi station of Harbin–Suifenhe Railway for one year. In spring 1939, I was transferred to Mudanjiang station as captain. In 1941, two captains were transferred to the station, one of them was Pengge Li and another one was Sun [name forgotten]. Pengge Li was a good man. He did not talk much and maybe was not keen on making friends.

In winter 1941, around the new year, when I was still captain, I heard that Pengge Li was arrested by the Japanese and his condition was unknown. In March 1942, I was transferred to station assistant in Mudanjiang. One day, an older Chinese woman came to the station, and I found that she was the mother of Pengge Li. She cried hard and asked if I knew where her son was who had not come home for a long time. His salary was stopped, and it was hard to maintain the family. She asked me for help. So, I asked Teiichi Hayashi [a Japanese man], the station manager, for information. Hayashi told me to ask the old woman to leave first, and he would tell. I sent the old woman home and asked Hayashi about Li.

Hayashi said, 'Pengge Li was killed by a secret agent in Harbin, because he drew the map of Mudanjiang airport and gave it to the Soviets. That Soviet agent was arrested in Harbin and revealed the name of Pengge Li. After his arrest, Li admitted the drawing was his and then he was killed.' Hayashi continued, 'tell her to find a way to go home.' I told the old woman the truth and helped her to collect money to go home. I posted a 'donation' notice at the Mudanjiang station and asked people to donate money for an old woman to go home. Later on, the money was collected and sent to the old woman. The old woman went home with the money.

According to the narrative, Teiichi Hayashi said, 'Pengge Li was executed by shooting in Harbin since he sent information to a Soviet secret agency.' However, the Jilin Provincial Archives kept another piece of information about special transfer that told a different story: on July 28, 1941, Kanto *Kempeitai* signed an order command sending Pengge Li and the other people as 'Soviet spies' to Harbin *Kempeitai*. The special transfer document of Harbin *Kempeitai* is number 605.[5]

In 1998, the 'name list of victims of special transfer by Unit 731' was released to media. Fengqin Li saw the news and visited the Unit 731 Museum in 2006 and saw her father's name, Pengge Li. Fengqin Li, then sixty-five years old, learned about her father for the first time. Since Li was a posthumous child who never met her father, I cannot imagine how much pain she suffered.

In 2011, the International Center for Unit 731 Research of the Harbin Academy of Social Sciences organised to 'revisit former places for victims of special transfer'. We went to Mudanjiang Railway Station to seek clues about her father. In 2012, the death of Pengge Li caused by the Japanese was confirmed. The Jilin Provincial government issued a martyr certificate for Pengge Li, which now hangs on the wall at Fengqin Li's home. This must be comfort for Li's family.

Story of Mudanjiang Information Station

In 1951, the former manager of Mudanjiang information station, Keren Zhuang , read an article in the magazine *Xinguancha*. The article confirmed 'Material of the case of former Japanese Army in preparing and producing bacterial weapons' that Zhiying Zhu, Dianxing Wu, and Chaoshan Sun were specially transferred to Unit 731. In 1992, the first curator of Unit 731 Museum Xiao Han heard about the information and interviewed Keren Zhuang in Beijing.

I have little material on this International Anti-Imperialism Information Organisation (国际反帝情报组织), therefore, it is hard to explain and comment about the organisation and its content. Basically, the International Anti-Imperialism Information Organisation was led by the Soviet Union Far East Information Organisation.

According Keren Zhuang:

> This 'international anti-imperialism information organisation' was set up in 1932. The leader was Wang Dongzhou and vice-leader was Yang Zuoqing. This organisation was set up to collect military information about the Japanese Army, organise anti-Japanese guerrillas and to destroy Japanese military facilities. I was responsible for Harbin and Mudanjiang information stations and mainly transmitted information to the Soviet Union Far East Information Organisation at Khabarovsk Krai.[6]

The stories of Zhiying Zhu, Dianxing Wu, and Enrui Jing are based on the interview with Xiao Han. In 1992, Xiao Han interviewed the witnesses, including Lanzhi Jing (wife of Zhiying Zhu), Guijie Long (wife of Huizhong Zhang), Xilin Jing (son of Enrui Jing), and Keren Zhuang (former manager of Mudanjiang Information Station). The interviews are kept in the Unit 731 Museum Archives.

The Stories of Zhiying Zhu and Lanzhi Jing

Lanzhi Jing was born in 1922 in Wangkui, Heilongjiang, and married Zhiying Zhu in 1938. He was a woodworker employed at Mudanjiang train station, but he was secretly working as an intelligence agent for the Soviet Union. On 16 July 1941, Zhiying Zhu was arrested by the Mudanjiang *Kempeitai* along with Huizhong Zhang, Dianxing Wu, Chaoshan Sun, and Enrui Jing (uncle of Lanzhi Jing). As anti-Japanese spies, they were all 'special transferred' to Unit 731 for human experimentation. None of them survived.

According to Lanzhi Jing:

> On July 17, 1941, as I was making dinner, a few Japanese *Kempeis* came into my home and searched around. They did not find anything. The Japanese asked me, 'What does Zhiying Zhu do? Where is the radio?' I said, 'Zhiying Zhu works at the railway, and I did not see any radio.' Later, the Japanese took me with their jeep to Mudanjiang *Kempeitai* compound. In the detention room, I saw Guijie Long, wife of Huizhong Zhang, and her two children. The next morning, *Kempeis* took me to a small house. They removed all my clothes, and asked me 'What does Zhiying Zhu do? What kind of activity does he do?' while whipping me. I said, 'he was a woodworker at the station. Besides going to work, I did not see him do anything else.' The Japanese continued, 'He is in anti-Japanese intelligence. Didn't you know what he does?' I said, 'I am a housewife. I really do not know anything. After the trial, the next morning,

the Japanese took me to the trial room on the second floor. Zhiying Zhu knelt in front of me with his clothes all removed and blood all over his face, like he just been tortured. The enemies hit me and interrogated me at the same time. Zhiying Zhu said in anger, 'Stop hitting her. She really knew nothing about it. All the activities were done by myself. Talk to me about anything.'[7]

Lanzhi Jing was imprisoned and released after one week. It was the last time Jing saw Zhiying Zhu. No one knew what life Zhiying Zhu had had all these years. Until 1995, with the help of Sino-Japanese grassroots organisation, Lanzhi Jing visited Tokyo, Japan, and revealed the truth about Zhiying Zhu and Enrui Jing .

She sued the Japanese Government, but the case was rejected by the Tokyo District Court. In 2005, I visited Lanzhi Jing for the first time. She was bedridden, and I could not hear her clearly. Later, she died with regrets (see Fig. 17).

The Stories of Huizhong Zhang and Guijie Long

Huizhong Zhang was born in April 1910 in Rongguan Village at Heihuazi, Dengta, of Liaoning Province, and learned tailoring in Shenyang in 1924. He was a worker in an arsenal at Shenyang in 1927 and joined the Chinese Communist Party the same year. He began to collect information about the Japanese in 1932 and became a photographer in Jinzhou the following year. In 1935, he studied at the Russian Military Academy in the Soviet Union and later studied radio waves in a university in the Moscow countryside. He was codenamed Alex and his number was '41'. He graduated in 1937, returned to Harbin, and married Guijie Long. In 1939, the Zhangs went to Mudanjiang where Zhang started work at Lushun Machinery as a fitter. There, Zhang secretly set up the Mudanjiang Information Station for the purpose of information collection. His direct supervisor was Keren Zhuang .

Guijie Long assisted Huizhong Zhang in sending and receiving telegrams. She recalled the day her husband was arrested:

Monday of the first week, Tuesday of the second week, Wednesday of the third week and Thursday of the fourth week of each month were the days we sent and received telegrams usually from 12 a.m. to 2 a.m. Each took about 20 minutes.

At midnight July 16, 1941, Zhang was working on telegrams at home. There were a lot telegrams to send and receive. The password codes took four pages. He worked from 12 a.m. until 2 a.m. to finish. I put the password code back, and Huizhong Zhang put away the radio in the box for horse feed and went to bed afterward. When we were about to fall asleep, there was huge noise in the backyard. I looked through the curtain and saw a lot of Japanese soldiers near the wall. I knew something bad happened. I woke Huizhong Zhang up and wrapped him with blankets as I knew there was not enough time to escape.

A Japanese soldier with a gun came through the north gate. He came inside the house and searched. He asked me, 'Where is the man?' I replied, 'at work!' 'Where does he work?' 'At the railway.'

The soldier searched the other rooms and Huizhong Zhang jumped from the window. Later, a Japanese soldier holding the radio entered the house. He put the radio on the kang and asked me, 'What is this?' 'I don't know.' Where is it from?' 'I picked it up from north of the railway,' I said loudly.

Huizhong Zhang was caught and taken away by the soldiers who were going to take me, too. When I went to get my child with me, I found a paper marked with password code on my child's blanket that had dropped out of the wooden box. Luckily, the soldier did not see it. I covered it with my body and slipped it inside the diaper and carried my baby. The Japanese soldier sent me to my neighbour Wei's home. They did not follow me to the room but directed me outside the house. I put the paper with password code under the blanket. A while later, one *Kempei* came and interrogated me.

'What is your name?'

'Guijie Long.'

'How old are you?'

'26 years old.'

'How many people in your family?'

'Four persons.'

'What is the name of your husband?'

'Huizhong Zhang.'

'What does he do?'

'He works with the railway carriage.'

'Where are you two from?'

'From Shenyang three years ago.'

'Where did the radio come from?'

'Picked up.'

'From which location?'

'From the north of the railway.'

They questioned me while hitting me at the same time. I was holding my child who was scared to cry. Japanese soldiers took away my child and hit me on my eye. They also choked my neck, and I fainted. When I woke up, I was guarded by two soldiers. They put handcuffs on my hands and sent me to the Mudanjiang *Kempetiai*. My two children were also sent to the *Kempeitai*. The oldest was only two years old and the younger one was just four months. We were sent to a temporary detention room. I held my children and wept in the corner near the window. I sat on the cold concrete floor, and because of the tiredness, I slept on the floor. At night, a Japanese soldier gave me a rice ball as dinner. I shared a large bite with my older child. He cried hard while he was eating. The younger kid was also crying nonstop.

The next morning, the soldiers took me to the backyard of the *Kempeitai*. They asked me to stand still. I heard Huizhong Zhang yelling from the second floor where he was being tortured. At around 10 a.m., the soldiers took me to another room. One

Japanese was sitting opposite me and there was a Chinese translator next to him. A bald-head Japanese soldier was recording.

The Japanese asked, 'Why didn't you say there is a radio at your home? When did the radio arrive?' I said, 'Just few days ago.' The Japanese asked, 'Where did the radio come from?' I said, 'I have no idea. I don't dare ask him. He would hit me whenever I asked. He always hit me.'

The Japanese said, 'Now you don't have to be afraid. Just tell whatever you know. What is the use of the radio?' I replied, 'I do not know.'

The translator came over and used two pencils to pinch my fingers. I screamed, and my two children were scared into crying again. The Japanese continued to ask, 'Where is the radio from?'

I replied, 'I do not know. I did not dare ask him. He told me if I keep asking him about his stuff, he will kill me and my kids. I am so scared of him. I always want to divorce him.'

After a week of suffering, the Japanese soldiers released me.

One evening two months later, the deputy captain of Mudanjiang *Kempeitai*, Ichiki Hasegawa, and Shiren Liu came to my home. They informed me that Huizhong Zhang and Zhiying Zhu were sent to Changchun. A few days before mid-autumn festival, Lanzhi Jing and I went to Changchun *Kempeitai* where one of the *Kempei* told us that they were sent to Harbin *Kempeitai*. We went to Harbin afterward, and we did not hear anything about them.[8]

Human Experimentation: Medical Ethics and Medical Crimes of Unit 731

From its beginning in 1933 until 1945, Unit 731 conducted inhumane and unethical human experiments to benefit Japan's biochemical warfare against China.

A huge number of Chinese, Russians, and Koreans were subjected to experiments, including living dissection, bacterial infections, and frostbite experiments. For 'the nation, scientific research and the development of the medical field', Unit 731 tortured and killed innocent citizens without consequence. After the war, the International Military Tribunal for the Far East ignored these grave war crimes. Until now, many Japanese leaders have chosen to forget these war crimes.

The Japanese doctors and researchers were exempted from responsibility for their acts. Furthermore, after the war, the perpetrators enjoyed privileges and prestigious job offers and became high-ranking officials in Japanese military departments and educational institutions, including high-status universities.

A number of them used data and statistics collected during experimentation in Unit 731 as material for their personal research through which they obtained doctoral degrees. They received offers of professorships and assistant professorships, and a number of them opened their own private hospitals and medical companies with their medical knowledge from Unit 731. These men did not regret their cruel behaviour at Unit 731 and enjoyed relatively stable and luxurious lives after the war.

Thanks to their reputed status in Japanese society, the human experimentation during the Second World War and medical war crimes committed by them while in the Japanese army were either covered up or ignored by the public.

It is time for Japan's medical field to take responsibility and expose these war crimes and the inhumane acts at Unit 731.

Secrets Within Secrets

When Unit 731 moved to Harbin from Tokyo in 1933, it set up Dong Man Jail (東滿大獄) at Beiyinhe of Wuchang to incarcerate anti-Japanese and ordinary citizens for experimentation. Construction of this jail marked the beginning of thirteen years of human experimentation by the Japanese.

Death Factory: The Square Quarter

In 1938, Unit 731 included in its headquarters design the Square Quarter, a core human experimentation venue, and a special jail to hold victims. The Square Quarter consisted of four three-storey buildings of 150 metres long and 100 metres wide. The special jail enclosed within the Square Quarter was made up of two two-storey buildings with capacity of up to 400 people. Unit 731 maintained close connections with the Kanto Army, the Japanese police, the Security Bureau, and other covert agencies to secure smooth transportation of captives used for human experimentation.

In preparing for experimentation, Unit 731 set up two sub-branches: a bacterial research division and a bacterial experiment division. These two sub-branches were mainly established for the creation and testing of bacteria before use on humans. Within the bacteria research division, there were sub-classes using the supervisor's name. For example, the 'Takahashi Class' was responsible for plague and the 'Minato Class' for Malaria. Unit 731 conducted experiments and research on more than fifty kinds of germs and viruses. Moreover, outside the Square Quarters there were facilities to manufacture poisonous gas, to conduct experiments on living humans, and to store these gas products and other protective devices (see Fig. 18).

Death Sequence Number of *Maruta*

Unit 731's Square Quarter and the special jail were the axis of human experimentation, as well its darkest secret. Captives there were experimental objects without basic human rights. They did not have a name, occupation, age, or background, only a three-digit number. They became '*marutas*' (Japanese for logs). When *marutas* arrived at the special jail, they were provided with food, drink, and exercise to keep them fit and healthy. Whenever a laboratory needed testers for experiments, they would select a healthy inmate and wrote their sequence number on a blackboard. Each number was a human life.

Regarding the number of *marutas*, the head of the First Division of Unit 731, Major General Nagakawa Kiyoshi, gave the following statement in the Khabarovsk Trial: 'Between 1940 and 1945, more than 3,000 people were killed by bacterial infection in the murder factory. For the number of people killed before 1940, I am not sure.'[1] Human experimentation had been carried out for a long time, its scale was large, and Japanese troops destroyed almost all the official documents regarding the experimentation when they retreated from Harbin. Records of 1933 to 1938 remain undiscovered, but from the oral narrative of former Japanese soldiers, it is confirmed that more than 3,000 people died in experimentation.

Death Laboratories

Unit 731 carried out large-scale human experimentation on war refugees, local labourers, peasants, craftspeople, men, women, and children. The experiments varied from live dissection, bacterial infection, frostbite, and poison gas to airborne infection, medical experiments, sub-dermal injections, and bombing.

Unimaginable Cruelty: Live Human Dissection

Until 731 staff dissected men, women, children, and even infants. The Japanese would not use the anaesthetics of *maruta* when they were in the process of dissection. The subjects were gagged, and their head, legs, and arms were tied with ropes on the operating table, where dissection materials were prepared.

Oral Narrative of an Old Soldier

Yoshio Tamura (田村良雄) of the youth class of Unit 731 revealed what he witnessed:

> One morning, a Chinese was planned to be the tester for dissection whether he was dead or alive. I put disinfectant on his body, head and neck. The face of that Chinese turned purple, and blood dropped to the floor from the stretcher. Oki shouted, 'Two camphor solutions!' and pointed two fingers at me which he ordered me to inject [into the Chinese patient]. The Chinese, who was tied by his legs and arms, suddenly opened his eyes wide after the injection of camphor. He looked as if he would like to see what was happening. He turned his head with tear-filled eyes. He looked at the ceiling. Hososhima used his hand to touch the neck of the Chinese, and he put the scalpel on it. Blood came out from the man's neck as his head turned left and right non-stop. Hososhima used the back of the scalpel to touch his heart and shouted, 'Two camphor solutions!' followed by a final cut in the Chinese's neck. The Chinese left his last word '*gui zi!*' ['evil!']. Hososhima used scalpels to cut from the upper stomach to the lower stomach, and from the lower stomach back to the chest of the Chinese. [He] used a chainsaw to cut his chest bones and finally showed all the viscera. After 20 minutes, the Chinese's body was chopped and the flesh was displayed on the surgery table with blood…[2]

Oral Narrative of Head of Military Police

Torao Yoshifusa, former Section Chief of the third section of the Kwantung Army *Kempeitai*, confessed after the war that he accompanied the commander-in-chief of the Kwantung Army *Kempeitai*, Major General Hara Mamoru, to inspect Unit 731.
Yoshifusa Taro said:

> … we walked about three metres along a corridor, and arrived at a dissecting room after turning left. As we were looking, three Japanese military surgeons immediately

stood and saluted when they saw Unit Chief Ishii. Ishii said, 'resume working,' they resumed what they were doing. A corpse was displayed on a dissection table at the centre of the space, still bleeding and each rib was clearly visible. Its skull was open; the brain fell to the left side of the body. Its hands and legs were fragmented, scattered at the right corner of the room. That bloody odour filled the room; even we, wearing face masks, felt nausea. Shirō Ishii sneered, 'Working here requires courage, but some military surgeons became madmen!'[3]

Living Teenager Dissected

When Unit 731 staff conducted vivisection, they exercised the so-called 'education and training' policy that allowed trainee doctors to observe. Nakaichi Kasuga , a military policeman of Unit 731, confessed an occasion when a Chinese teenager was dissected:

That Chinese teenager, not over 12 or 13 years old, was nude on an operating table. His body was wiped with alcohol instead of general anaesthesia. Holding a scalpel and approaching the teenager, Employee K from Tanabe Class, whose members stood around the table, cut his chest in a Y-shape. Gore squelched from a haemostat, and white fat was revealed. K expertly took out each organ such as intestines, pancreas, liver, kidney and stomach from the sleeping teenager and threw them into drums. Someone immediately picked up the organs from the drums and placed them into a large glass container filled with formalin solution in advance and closed the container with a cover. Kōzō Okamoto, the leader of the dissection class, while dissecting the body and explaining to the class, was putting bloody organs into specimen bottles. Afterward, the trainee doctors swarmed the body, and each tried to practise dissection.[4]

Scalpel Used on Prisoners

Among the ethically controversial actions of Unit 731, military surgeons acted even more controversially: they used other Japanese members of Unit 731 as vivisection material. In *A History of the Crimes of Unit 731 of the Japanese Army*, co-written by Xiao Han and Peilin Xin, Yoshio Tamura confessed:

This dissection was strictly confidential. Sudō Yoshio was an employee of the First division, the Fourth department, who was infected with bubonic plague because of the production of plague bacteria. In a dissection room of the special class, Hasoya the technician was conducting vivisection, and I was the assistant of Hasoya. Hasoya first dissected a Chinese. Immediately after this, Suzuki ordered to dissect Sudō Yoshio, who was dying and was transferred to the dissection room. Naked Sudō Yoshio was moved to a dissection table by members of the special class. A few days previously, Sudō had still been interested in talking about women, but now he was as thin as a rake, with many purple spots over his body. A large area of scratches on his chest were bleeding. He painfully cried and breathed with difficulty.

I sanitised Sudō's whole body with disinfectant. Because of the effect of the disinfectant, Sudō became conscious and opened his blank eyes to look around. Whenever he moved, a rope around his neck tightened. After Suzuki carefully checked Sudō's whole body, he ordered dissection to begin. I handed a scalpel to Hosoya, and Hosoya, reversing the scalpel, went towards Sudō and handed the scalpel to Uno. Uno touched Sudō's stomach skin, his hands slightly shaking. At this moment, Suzuki hysterically shouted, 'Hurry up!' Reversely gripping the scalpel, Uno pierced Sudō's upper stomach and sliced downwards. Blood flowed into a pool on the dissection table. Shouting 'Brute!' Sudō died with this last word.[5]

Treated Like Animals:
Oral Treatment, Injection and Infection Experiments

After the Second World War, Dr Norbert Fell of Fort Detrick, US Army, investigated Shirō Ishii, Tomosada Masuda, Junichi Kaneko, Ryōichi Naitō, and others in Japan. On 20 June 1947, Fell submitted a 'Brief Summary of New Information about Japanese BW Activities', commonly known as the Fell Report.

The Fell Report details human experiments with anthrax, bubonic plague, and cholera conducted by Unit 731 through various infection methods, including oral medication and injection. It cites all data of human experiments conducted by Unit 731, which tested for the lowest infective dose and the lethal dose of various bacteria. It includes the following:

Inserted rubber tubes into noses of three experimental subjects. These three people were all infected after inhaling 0.1 mg of bacteria.

The median lethal dose of *Bacillus anthracis* through subcutaneous injection was 10mg while it was 50 mg through oral intake. The death rate of those who received the subcutaneous injection was 66%, 90% for those who received the oral intake, and 100% for those who had open wounds. The median lethal dose of *Yersinia pestis* through subcutaneous injection was 10–6 mg while it was 0.1 mg through oral intake. The infection rate was 80% if breathing for ten seconds with 5 mg/m³ of the concentration. The incubation period of direct infection was generally three to five days, and one would die three to seven days later following fever.[6]

Yatarō Ueda had been an assistant participating in a comparative experiment of *Yersinia pestis* infection. In 1956, at a management station of war criminals in Fushun, he said:

… at first, five experimental subjects were injected 0.1g *Yersinia pestis*, another five for 0.2 g, another five for 0.3 g, and the first comparison table was created based on observation results. Secondly, five experiment subjects were embedded with 0.1 g, 0.2 g and 0.3 g *Yersinia pestis* respectively, and the second comparison table was created based on observation results. The third comparison table was based on five experimental subjects who received oral intake of 0.1 g, 0.2 g and 0.3 g *Yersinia pestis* respectively.[7]

That forty-five people were employed for one experiment on *Yersinia pestis* suggests that the number and scale of experiments conducted by Unit 731 were quite high and large. These lives were ignored as human beings. To those military surgeons, *maruta* were ideal experiment material through which they could obtain more accurate and more detailed data than they could achieve with other methods. This obviously violated the principle that medical research should be for the benefit of humanity.

Victims Tied to Stakes: Bomb Experiments

To conduct large-scale human experiments in the field, Unit 731 set up the Chengzigou Experimental Field at its headquarters in Pingfang; the Anda Special Experimental Field (now Anda city in Heilongjiang Province); and the Taolaizhao Experimental Field (in what is currently Fuyu city in Jilin Province). Memoirs of veterans of Unit 731, the Arvo Thompson Report, the Thomas Inglis Report, and the Fell Report also record that Unit 731 tested germ bombs on human bodies in the field.

Unit 731 conducted both field and laboratory experiments with *Yersinia pestis* as an agent of germ warfare. In his report, Fell notes:

> … sprayed with the bacteria by a flight flying low, an experimental subject was jailed in a room in a *Yersinia pestis* experiment, who would be infected for 30% to 100% with at least 60% death rate. In an explosion experiment using UJI ceramic bombs with a detonating cord in which fleas were mixed with sand, approximately 80% of fleas were still alive after the explosion. In a 10-m² room of ten experimental subjects, eight were infected by flea bites in an explosion experiment, and six of them died eventually.[8]

Unit 731 also filled bombs with anthrax, *Yersinia pestis*, and glandes bacteria.
The Inglis Report states:

> … tied experimental subjects wearing helmet and body armour on stakes, and detonated Ishii ceramic germ bombs by both throwing and placing at particular places. In one experiment, of 15 living humans as experimental subjects, six were killed by the explosion, four were injured and infected with anthrax. These four infected persons died later. In another experiment of Ishii ceramic germ bombs, of ten people, four died of respiratory infection who were located at distance of 25 m from the explosion spot.[9]

Unit 731 also used animals such as horses, cows, and sheep in field experiments. The Thompson Reports states: '… in an experiment of germ bombs placed 15m height from the ground, a bomb was detonated. Animals were grazing downwind for one to two hours, and almost 70% of horses and 90% of sheep died.[10]

Detailed Report: Frostbite Experiment

Unit 731 specially established the Frostbite Studies Section and the Frostbite Laboratory to conduct experiments, produce dried bacteria, and study prevention and treatment methods of frostbite.

Materials, such as 'On Frostbite Experiment', an article by Hisato Yoshimura, head of the Frostbite Studies Section, have been found and publicised, and the entire process of frostbite experiment has also been publicly disclosed.[11] According to the article, it was identified that data presented by Hisato Yoshimura was based on human experiments. Hisato Yoshimura was not put on trial after the Second World War, but published *The Gist of Medical Physiology* and *The Theory of pH and its Examination Method* based on his research experiences and data obtained in Unit 731, attaining high social status in the Japanese medical field and serving in public positions, including as vice-chancellor of Kyoto Prefectural University of Medicine.

Gokuhi Chūmōgun Tōki Eisei Kenkyū Seiseki (*Highly Confidential Results of Hygiene Research in Winter by Mongolia Garrison Army*) was released in Japan in the 1990s, further confirming parts of the historical facts that not only was Unit 731 involved in frostbite experiments, but several other Epidemic Prevention and Water Purification Departments of the Japanese military also actively participated in this war crime (see Fig. 19).

According to *Gokuhi Chūmōgun Tōki Eisei Kenkyū Seiseki*, in March 1941, the Epidemic Prevention and Water Purification Department of the Northern China Area Army and the Epidemic Prevention and Water Purification Department of the Mongolia Garrison Army jointly conducted frostbite experiments in the field at west Sonid in Xilingol League. Eight Chinese subjects were used for the experiment: Chun Liu (aged twenty-seven), Chun Pan (aged twenty-two), Fu Gao (aged thirty-three), Guan Xia (aged fifteen), Bai Gao (aged forty-nine), Gui Hao (aged thirty-five), Yi Zhang (aged twenty-one), and Yuan Chen (aged thirty-eight). Either their surname or given name were intentionally hidden by the Japanese military.

Records show the aim of this experiment was 'investigation for hygienic demand during the cold period when fighting on Inner Mongolia grassland and for the next battle'. It was jointly organised by various Epidemic Prevention and Water Purification Departments of the Japanese military. In the process of the human frostbite experiment, they observed pathological changes and related characteristics at intervals, recorded corresponding data, and took photographs on site for better documentation of results (see Figures 20 and 21).[12]

Detailed data on frostbite experiments was contained in this information. From the record:

From 6:30 to 9:30 on February 6, 1941, the outside temperature is minus 24 to 27 degrees. Wind speed was five meters per second. Human subjects were placed supine on stretchers in order to observe their frostbite situation. The Japanese army divided them into five types: those in bare hands, in wet socks or wet gloves, and those wearing smaller military boots. Some subjects were over-drinking, fasting or had been given atropine.[13] The following conclusions were reached:

1. Bare hands: frostbite occurred within 5 to 25 minutes.

2. Used gloves: frostbite occurred after 20 minutes, some occurred after 3 hours.

3. Wore military boots: frostbite occurred after 1 hour.

4. Used anti-cold shoe: frostbite occurred after 1.5 hours, but most occurred after 3 hours.

5. Wore wet gloves and wet socks: frostbite occurred 50% faster than in dry conditions. Frostbite of hands happened faster than of feet. It might be because of the anti-cold shoes.

6. Wore too small military boots: frostbite occurred 50% less than with normal size boots.

7. Frostbite happened slower than bare hands (25 minutes) and with wet socks (1 hour 40 minutes) during fasting condition. It is not understandable.

8. Frostbite happened slower than bare hands (30 minutes) with wet socks (20 minutes) and with anti-cold shoes and socks (1 hour) during drunk condition. It varied by person.

9. Took 5 units of atropine before frostbite experiment, frostbite occurred 1.5 hours with temperature of minus 14 degrees with wind speed of 0.7 meters per second and bare hands. When in bare feet, frostbite occurred in toes after 35 minutes.

10. For frostbite treatment, it took 25 minutes to 2 hours for friction. To apply friction on frostbite, cloths were used for friction to make the skin red, soft and warm. After the first treatment, there will be blisters within 8 hours and bigger blisters within 24 hours.[14]

After the eight Chinese subjects were tortured in frostbite experiments, they suffered vivisection and the Japanese Army photographed the victims during this. Recognition was made of the victims for 'giving their lives to contribute to medical advances for humanity'.

Poison Gas Experiments on Humans

The bacterial and vivisection experiments conducted by Unit 731 are known to the public; however, poison gas experiments are little known. I visited the National Archives and Records Administration II and read the record: Unit 731 established laboratories for poison gases replete with departments of research, production, experiments, and prevention. The laboratories defined different types of poison gases and tested and produced gas masks and protective suits.

The Ishii-style poison gas analyser, Ishii-style anti-poison gas medicine, and Ishii-style testing paper and disinfectants for poison gas were simultaneously invented at these laboratories. Based upon the large number of gas masks left in the former site of Unit 731, as well as the size of gas laboratories and gas storage rooms and also the official records in the US, Unit 731 was not a secret agency dedicated solely to bacterial warfare research, it was concerned with research on poisonous weapon invention at the same time (see Fig. 22).

Diary of Lt-Gen. Endo, Vice-Chief of Staff of the Kanto Army

Unit 731 conducted large-scale poison gas experiments, and used vivisection during that process and during poison gas weapons production. The earliest human poison gas experiment took place in 1933.

In *Shogun no yuigon: Endo Saburo nikki*, Miyataki writes:

> On October 16, Thursday, sunny. At 8:30 am, Colonel Ando and Lieutenant Colonel Tachibara and I went for observation at the experimental field of transportation division. The second class were experiments on poisonous gases and venom. The first class was experiment with electricity. Each class used two 'thieves' in the experiments. The people were experimented on in the gas laboratory, one was treated with phosgene (poisonous gas) for five minutes and was infected with pneumonia. The subject's life was in danger, even more serious than yesterday, although there were still signs of life. Another one was injected with 15 ml of potassium cyanate and passed out after about 20 minutes.[15]

Report of Human Experimentation Using Poison Gas Discovered in Japan

In 1983, Professor Takao Matsumura of Keio University discovered a report of human experimentation with poison gas. 'The Harm to Skin Incurred by Yellow Paintball and General Clinical Observation' consists of forty-seven pages with three maps and was written by Lt-Col. Ikeda Naeo of the Kamo Division.[16] Kamo Division was the preliminary name of Unit 731. It recorded experiments conducted from 7–10 September 1940 at Mudanjiang on twenty people placed in simulated shelters, trenches, and sitting rooms. Test subjects were attacked with mustard gas in order to observe reactions and collect data.

The aforementioned report recorded:

> The gun shot 1,800 mustard bombs on area one and 3,200 on area two. Area three was shot with 4,800 mustard bombs. There were five testers at area one. Their numbers were 287, 280, 296, 294 and 376. Area two contained six testers, and their numbers were 256, 464, 468, 490, 499 and 513. Area three had nine testers whose numbers were 303, 485, 486, 372, 358, 259, 449, 375 and 265.[17]

Following the attacks, observation was done after four hours, twelve hours, twenty-four hours, forty-eight hours, and seventy-two hours. The symptoms of the testers, their skin, eyes, and condition of respiratory and digestive organs, were well-recorded in a detailed list. This was the method used by Unit 731 on *marutas*: victims known by three-digits instead of names.

The Struggle of Marutas

Although their victims were only numbers to the staff of Unit 731, stories of their resistance were recorded in the novel *The Devil's Feast*, written by Seiichi Morimura. The following is an excerpt:

It was early June in 1945, on a sunny morning. There were two Russian '*marutas*' kept in the No.7 prison. One of them said he did not feel well and lay down on the floor. Another informed the guard that 'the person in this room looks unusual', and he was with the sick cellmate with handcuffs on his hands. The members of Unit 731 saw this as an unusual condition in the prison so they went entered the cell. The Russian lying on the floor suddenly sprang up and knocked the guard down. The two Russians opened their handcuffs, took the keys and opened the other cells one by one, while yelling 'Run outside, run!' The entrance of the special prison, however, was blocked by a metal door, and the rest of Unit 731 staff were inside the prison with guns. Some *marutas* who were not able to escape, including Russian and Chinese, were walking the corridors and kept yelling and shouting.

Members of Unit 731 yelled at the prisoners: 'Go back to the cells or we will shoot you. Go back quickly. Don't shout'. One Russian shouted to the members of Unit 731: 'You are threatening us with guns. But we are not afraid … Japanese are cowards. Release us now. We'd rather be killed by you now than used as experimental objects like guinea pigs'.

This Russian held up his fist, hit the fences and kept yelling loudly. One Chinese in black clothes yelled at the staff of Unit 731 and beat his chest strongly at the same time. The confident shouts and angry faces made the members of Unit 731 angry. One of them shot a Russian to death. The rebellion by *marutas* was suppressed.[18]

One of the eyewitnesses on staff at Unit 731 recalled:

When I remember the words of that Russian, it was a wish from the deepest part of a heart of a man whose freedom was taken away. But at that time, I could not understand his emotion. I was thinking *marutas* are not human. How can we be looked down on by them? How can they rebel? Before his death, the powerful attitude of his protest against the guns left an impressive image on us. The Russian was knocked down by a bullet, and we used bullets to shut their mouths up. But spiritually we were all lost in front of the *marutas* who had no freedom and no weapons. At that time, we understood in our hearts that justice was not on our side.[19]

Human Experimentation with Anthrax and Glanders

In November 2011, I visited the Science, Technology and Business Division of the Library of Congress to search for Unit 731 material. With the assistance of Ms Tomoko Y. Steen, I received two reports on human experimentation written by a member of Unit 731: 'Report A of Human Experimentation by Anthrax' and 'Report G of Human Experimentation by Glanders'. These two reports are the core information of the secret deal between the US Army and Unit 731 in the early period after the end of the Second World War (see Fig. 23).

30 Cases of Human Experimentation with Anthrax: Report 'A'

'A' refers to anthrax, the abbreviation used by Unit 731. The report is 406 pages in English, with 'Dugway Proving Ground Technical Library, May 6, 1960' on the cover.

Pages 292 to 311 concern changes to adrenal glands. In this section, microfilms No. M325 and No. M54, both marked 'Detrick', are indicated. Fort Detrick, Fredericksburg, Maryland, is where the US Army conducted secret research on bacterial warfare. It proves Report 'A' was kept at the Detrick base and that the army conducted human experimentation with anthrax (see Fig. 24).

Structure of Report 'A'

Report 'A' consists of two parts: a sixteen-page introduction including the details of the listed cases, and a micro investigation.

Report 'A' records thirty cases divided into three based on the source of infection: the first is skin infection, of which there is recorded one case; the second type is nine cases of oral infection; and the third is twenty cases of nasal respiratory infection. Report 'A' was originally written in Japanese before being translated by the US Army into English after the report was received from Unit 731.

The thirty case subjects were all adult males. Their information has been summarised into the following list:

Basic Information of Test Subjects in Report 'A'					
Sequence	Number	Gender	Age	Days of process	Source of infection
1	17	M	38	2	Oral infection
2	18	M	29	2	Oral infection
3	26	M	25	3	Oral infection
4	54	M	25	7	Skin infection
5	225	M	35	2	Oral infection
6	318	M	30	2	Oral infection
7	320	M	30	2	Oral infection
8	325	M	25	2	Oral infection
9	328	M	32	2	Oral infection
10	383	M	40	3	Oral infection
11	388	M	27	2	Nasal respiratory infection
12	389	M	25	3	Nasal respiratory infection
13	390	M	25	3	Nasal respiratory infection
14	393	M	34	4	Nasal respiratory infection
15	396	M	29	3	Nasal respiratory infection

16	397	M	27	4	Nasal respiratory infection
17	399	M	26	3	Nasal respiratory infection
18	400	M	32	3	Nasal respiratory infection
19	401	M	37	2	Nasal respiratory infection
20	403	M	34	3	Nasal respiratory infection
21	404	M	27	3	Nasal respiratory infection
22	405	M	27	3	Nasal respiratory infection
23	406	M	31	2	Nasal respiratory infection
24	407	M	28	3	Nasal respiratory infection
25	409	M	32	2	Nasal respiratory infection
26	410	M	27	3	Nasal respiratory infection
27	411	M	28	4	Nasal respiratory infection
28	412	M	27	3	Nasal respiratory infection
29	413	M	37	3	Nasal respiratory infection
30	414	M	29	2	Nasal respiratory infection

Interpretation and Analysis

Basic information about the victims, including name, occupation, birthplace, and life history, were excluded in the report. They became only numbers, with their gender and age kept as reference for experiments. The oldest victim was forty years old, and the youngest four victims were twenty-five years old. The average age of the victims was 29.88 years old and the average infection period was 2.88 days. Using microscopic examination, the Unit recorded in detail infections that occurred in heart, lung, tonsils, bronchi, throat, liver, stomach, spleen, kidneys, pancreas gland, adrenal gland, thyroid, testis, pituitary, brain, skin, lymph nodes, and other organs (see Fig. 25).

The condition of the nine orally infected victims recorded in Report 'A' was 'Through anthrax-infected food, the infected people died of serious oral infection and ascites bleeding'. The report described twenty cases of nasal respiratory infected victims 'a sudden outbreak of anthrax infection occurred in some cells. Twenty victims were infected through air transmittal. A few days later, they were found dead due to acute chest and abdomen symptoms. In the first phase, they suffered from acute tonsillitis. Anthrax went throughout the body and led to serious bleeding. Major spreading occurred at bronchus and mouth.'

21 Human Experimentation with Glanders: Report 'G'

Unit 731's Report 'G' (glanders) is 373 pages and makes mention of the twenty-one human subjects involved, divided into two parts: the first part is the introduction, including general information about all infected victims, their symptoms, and conditions. The second part is microscopic observation of the condition of infected organs including heart, lung, tonsils, bronchia and throat, liver, stomach, intestine, spleen, kidneys, pancreas, adrenal glands, thyroid, thymus, testis, pituitary gland, brain, skin, and lymph nodes (see Fig. 26).

Report 'G' noted the death of victims through four stages. In the first or acute period, there were eight human subjects whose numbers were 224, 180, 190, 16, 176, 178, and 229. One of the cases was missing a number. Some parts near the organs showed symptoms of septicaemia, but no obvious conditions were found. The second was a subacute period. There were seven cases, numbers 167, 50, 254, 85, 207, 221, and 193. Symptoms included acute systemic metastases at around the two-week mark, especially to the lungs, with frequent pleurisy bleeding. Due to systemic metastases, serious exudative lesions occurred in the lungs and liver. The third type was the sub-chronic period represented by three cases numbered 205, 146, and 152. The fourth was the chronic period involving three cases numbered 256, 727, and 731. Their symptoms included infection in lungs, livers, intestines, lymphs, kidneys, muscles, and thyroids due to serious systemic metastases.

Based on Reports 'A' and 'G' kept by the Library of Congress, as well as the current Chinese and Japanese literature, here are my conclusions:

Two reports in the Library of Congress are relatively complete reports on human experimentation and important evidence regarding Unit 731's conduct of it. They may be used for cross-checking against documents on special transportation kept by Heilongjiang Provincial Archives and Jilin Provincial Archives. These reports are written in English, along with the existing Chinese and Japanese documents, and have great significance in revealing the war crimes of Unit 731.

The two reports contain rich statistics, including information on sources of infection, days of infection, pathological changes in organs and causes of death. These data obtained by Unit 731 are valuable in research on infection with anthrax and glanders, vaccine production and disease prevention.

Through the analysis of the two reports, researchers may gain a better understanding of the way Unit 731 conducted medical research, and it further reveals evidence proving their war crimes through bacterial experiments.

Each case in the two reports is written and analysed after being carefully observed by microscope in order to generalise pathological changes, cause of infection and ratio of infection. From a medical perspective, these two reports are detailed reports of vivisection. Besides producing bacterial weapons and experiments, Unit 731 also conducted full-scale medical research for Japan's aggressive military, which is completely against medical ethics and humanity.

Conclusion and Reflection

Although the Second World War ended in 1945, many Japanese people still deny and distort the war crimes committed by Japan against humanity and human rights. The memories and history of the Second World War are common to both countries, and the perceptions of historical issues between China and Japan remain influential on bilateral relations today.

Japan's medical circle in the post-war period has not sufficiently faced and reflected on the medical war crimes committed during the war, but has chosen to be silent and evade as well as to deny and deceive.

Some civil organisations in Japan urge justice and truth, but in general, they have little impact on the mainstream of Japan's medical community. Regarding its cruel human experiments, medical crimes, and atrocities, Japan's medical community lacks introspection and reflection on 'the reason of state, human rights and medical ethics', and this attitude is also a miniature of post-war Japanese mainstream society, which evaded responsibility for the war and for distorting historical fact.

War and Medicine, an exhibition panel brochure prepared by The Research Society for 15 Years' War and Japanese Medical Science and Service, contains the following:

> The 'reflection from an original point of view' will never be possible without reflecting upon the morality of Japanese medicine during the early Showa period and the Fifteen Years' War to the following post-war period when medical science and practices in Japan began to develop and modernize. Above all, the participation of the Japan Medical Association (JMA) the Japanese Association of Medical Sciences (JAMS) in the Fifteen Years' War and the 'human experimentation' and 'vivisections' performed by Japanese medical scholars/doctors call out for our inevitable and sincere repentance, considering the inheritance of the post-war medicine from such practices.... During these 60 years, almost no commitment has been made to face this issue and the like seriously and to learn a lesson therefrom.[20]

In September 1947, medical associations of forty-five countries jointly organised The World Medical Association. Representatives noted members from Germany and Japan had committed atrocities during the Second World War, and therefore adopted a resolution that medical associations from Germany and Japan were required to submit an introspection announcement when they joined the Association.

In 1951, the Japan Medical Association joined the World Medical Association, having announced that 'as the representative institution of Japanese doctors, JMA, on this occasion, reprimands the violence inflicted upon the people of the enemy countries, and condemns the alleged and in a few cases actually performed cruelties on patients'.

War and Medicine stated: 'This statement, although the only official comment on these issues, is not yet oriented towards a serious reflection on the wartime behaviour of the Japanese medical profession, nor to a consequent reconsideration for the future of the ideal/morals of medical science and practice'.

In its persistence in evading these issues, Japan's medical community seems to look forward to forgetting those medical atrocities over time, to look forward to the moment that medical war criminals represented by the Unit 731 and their descendants will be relieved of being asked for introspection. Given the ambiguity concerning the atrocities, the statement by the Japan Medical Association in 1951 was no more than a false recognition and an indifferent promise to the general public in order to join the World Medical Association.

In his article, 'The Medical Crime in the Fifteen Years' War and Our Task Today', Shozo Azami, a Japanese scholar, says: '... the subordinate officers who follow the order of the superior officer are liable to punishment when they know it is against martial law and civil law.... Although the Nuremberg code had not yet been established at the time of the Fifteen Years' War, "never do harm to human life" is the basic principle of judgment for doctors and medical scientists'.[21]

In 2003, an American professor, Michael J. Franzblau, urged Japan's medical circle do genuine introspection on Unit 731, saying 'to look away from the Unit 731 issue is to degrade yourselves'.

At the end of his article, Shozo Azami writes:

What we demand from the present Japanese medical establishment is to reflect the fact that they have avoided facing squarely the medical crimes during the war, and to think deeply and seriously about what that fact implies ... after the disclosure of Unit 731 issues, the reason why Japanese medical scientists and doctors have still shielded them is probably related to the inferiority complex that they have kept the issues secret in their hearts. Why do they feel inferior? It is because they actually knew what the Ishii Unit was doing in the past, which was a public secret. If this is why they keep silent, then their silence is indeed a crime.[22]

On the seventieth anniversary of the end of the Second World War, the Department of Medicine of Kyushu University, Japan exhibited historical material about the vivisection of eight American pilots. Of those Japanese doctors who participated in the vivisection, five were sentenced to the death penalty, four to life imprisonment, and fourteen to imprisonment. However, as the Korean War broke out, the US military used excuses to release all the doctors, and not one was executed.

Given this background, there are two things we should consider: under what circumstances in the Cold War can Americans give up the spirit of humanism and its value? Can they exempt from trial and release war criminals if the criminals cruelly massacred people of their nationality?

The vivisection cases exhibited at Kyushu University were the first occasion that Japan's medical community displayed material on medical and ethical crimes committed during the Second World War on a large scale. It was not an unacceptable starting point. Indeed, it could be a beginning of honestly perceiving history, memory, and the future.

Bacteriological Warfare

Unit 731 planned and skilfully designed a fully-equipped base with all necessary facilities in the Pingfang area in Harbin. The base was built to prepare for bacteriological warfare. The Unit prepared and launched a series of outdoor field experimentations on bacterial bombs, bacterial vaccines, and bacteriological war strategy.

At the same time, the Japanese imported a large number of rats, mice, and rabbits as experimental objects used to spread bacteria along with insects such as fleas, lice, flies, and mosquitoes. These living creatures were infected with more than fifty kinds of bacteria, including plague, typhoid fever, anthrax, glanders, and tuberculosis, for research on bacteriological warfare.

Since the battles of Nomonhan in 1939, Unit 731 and all other similar units in Japan intensified their efforts in carrying out research and planning for bacteriological warfare on behalf of Imperial Japan. The quantity of the biochemical weapons and bacterial vaccines that were produced by Unit 731 alone would be sufficient to infect and eliminate the entire global population.

According to the current data at hand, Unit 731 and other units had indeed conducted large-scale bacteriological warfare in a vast expense of land in China, ranging from Hulunbuir of Inner Mongolia, Changchun in Jilin Province, Nong'an, and west of Shandong peninsula to upper Jiangxi, Guangfeng, Nanjing, Hangzhou, Ningbo, Quzhou, Jinhua, Yiwu, Yunhe, Jiangshan, Longyou, Lishui, Changsha, Changde, and west of Yunnan. All these communities suffered from widespread plague, cholera, and typhoid fever resulting in a high death rate. Japanese bacteriological warfare brought disaster to the Chinese population along with huge violations of the ecosystem as well as human societies. Although the war ended long ago, the harm and disaster remain.

Due to the high secrecy, members of Unit 731 and related units were able to evade the Tokyo trials with the cooperation of the US. Former members of the Unit chose not to reveal the truth, making the investigation process an extremely complicated task. In recent years, the US has begun to declassify material related to Japanese bacteriological warfare that allows researchers further avenues of investigation.

Research, Experimentation, and Choice of Bacteriological Weapons and Bacterial Vaccines

'Inglis's Report' by Thomas B. Inglis, 'Thompson's Report' by Arvo T. Thompson, 'Fell's Report' by Nobert Fell, and 'Hill's Report' by Edwin V. Hill recorded the details of bacteriological warfare and bacterial vaccines invented or developed by Unit 731.

Bacteria Bombs

From 1937 to 1942, Unit 731 invented at least 1,770 bacteria bombs (see Chart 1), including Model I, Model RO, Model U, Model GA, Older Model UJI, Model UJ150, Model JUI100, Model HA, Model SI, and the cluster bomb.

Chart 1: Details of Bacterial Bombs[1]			
Serial	Bomb	Quantity	Production Year
1	Model I	300	1937
2	Model RO	300	1937
3	Model U	20	1939
4	Model GA	50	1940
5	Older Model UJI	300	1938
6	Model UJ150	500	1940–1942
7	Model UJI100	300	1941–1942
8	Model HA	Unknown	Unknown
9	Model SI	Unknown	Unknown
10	Cluster Bomb	Unknown	Unknown

Of the ten types of bacterial bombs, UJ150 was the most frequently produced. The UJ150—also known as Model UJI—was built in a ceramic shell in Ishii style (Shirō Ishii, leader of Unit 731). Like the Ishii-style filter, UJ150 was invented and produced by Shirō Ishii. From 1940 to 1943, 500 Ishii-style ceramic bombs were produced. The quantity of fragments of UJ150 bombs found in the Unit 731 ruins—as well as the scale of the former factory (a five-storey building, with two kilns and four chimneys) located in Wanggang Village, Nangang, Harbin—indicate huge-scale production.

The chief aim of Unit 731 was to produce bombs with great lethality and destructive power that were easy to carry. From 1937 to 1942, at least ten kinds were tested. Information such as type of bombs, types of bacterial liquid, attack results, and production budgets were widely studied.

In Thompson's Report, Shirō Ishii claims these experiments did not follow official command and were medical research to prevent disease. However, based on current materials, the aim of producing bacteria bombs was to eventually initiate bacteriological warfare. The scale of design and experiments make it impossible that they were part of medical research for military purposes. The experimental data, statistics, and drawings from Inglis's Report and Thompson's Report confirm that Unit 731 was established for the purpose of bacteriological warfare research (see Fig. 27).

Bacterial Liquid

Regarding the records on the type of bacterial liquid invented by Unit 731, I referred to medical reports and academic articles written by former Unit 731 members as well as oral narratives collected by the US Army.

Oral Narratives of Former Soldiers

Army surgeon Tomoshisa Masuda, a core member of Unit 731, supporter of Shirō Ishii, the third division head of Unit 731 and the head of Unit 1644, was investigated by Sanders and Thompson of the US Army. Masuda submitted a report entitled 'Bacteriological Warfare' to the US Army on 15 December 1942. He believed four types of bacterial liquid could be used in warfare. One of them is bacteria, including plague, cholera, typhoid fever, dysentery, glanders, anthrax, brucellosis, tularaemia, tuberculosis, tetanus, gas gangrene, Botulinum toxin, diphtheria, *Staphylococcus*, *Streptococcus*, and meningococcal meningitis. The second was protozoa, such as Farber disease, relapsing fever, yaws, malaria, and kala-azar. The third type was rickettsia, such as typhus, typhus fever, and scrub typhus. The last type was viruses, such as dengue, yellow fever, smallpox, foot and mouth disease, rabies, and epidemic anaemia (see Fig. 29).[2]

Army surgeon Hojo Enryo, a supporter and assistant of Ishii, was a core member in the research epidemic prevention centre established by the School of Army Surgeons (Tokyo) in 1932. He was a member of the Japanese Medical Office and studied bacteriology at the Robert Koch Institute in Berlin, Germany. On 10 April 1947, Hojo was interrogated by the US Army and submitted his 1941 report 'About Bacteriological Warfare' in which he explained:

> The following bacteria can be used in bacteriological warfare. First is bacteria for human beings, including vibrio cholera, dysentery *Bacillus*, paratyphoid *Bacillus*, brucellosis, plague *Bacillus*, rabbit fever bacteria, salmonella, typhoid and yellow fever. The second type is for animals including anthrax, glanders, CBPP and foot and mouth disease. The third type is for plants, such as wheat *Puccinia*, *Mycovellosiella*, *Erwinia* and *Cercospora* for potatoes and other plants.[3]

Concluding Reports from the US Army

'Thompson's Report' recorded the narratives of Shirō Ishii and Masaji Kitano about the types of bacteria Unit 731 researched:

> ... typhoid and paratyphoid, dysentery, cholera, plague, pertussis, meningococcal meningitis vaccine and gonococcal. Toxin research was done to prevent gas gangrene, tetanus, diphtheria and scarlet fever. In order to prevent gas gangrene,

tetanus, diphtheria, scarlet fever, erysipelas, dysentery, *Streptococcus*, *Staphylococcus*, pneumonia, meningococcal meningitis and plague serum therapy was improved. Also, [Unit 731] conducted research on typhus, epidemic haemorrhagic fever, forest tick encephalitis, rabies, smallpox vaccine and bacteria vaccine.[4] [See Fig. 28.]

'Fell's Report' recorded nine types of bacteria used in human experimentation: anthrax, plague, typhoid, paratyphoid fever, paratyphoid 'B', dysentery, cholera, glanders, and epidemic haemorrhagic fever. The experiments included direct infection experiments, immunisation experiments, bomb tests, stability tests, and spray tests.

Hill interrogated twenty-two former members of Unit 731 and put his conclusions in 'Hill's Report'. In total, twenty-nine kinds of agents were researched by Unit 731.

Chart 2: Bacterial agents recorded in 'Hill's Report'[5]		
Serial	Type of Bacterial Agent	Interrogated Individuals
1	Typhoid	Kozo Akamoto, Seiwa Tanabe
2	Paratyphoid 'A' and 'B'	Unrecorded
3	Dysentery	Ueda Masaaki, Tomoshisa Masuda, Saburo Kojima, Seiwa Tanabe
4	Cholera	Tachiomaru Ishikawa, Kozo Okamoto
5	Plague	Shirō Ishii, Masahiro Takahashi, Kozo Okamoto, Tachiomaru Ishikawa
6	Anthrax	Masumi Ota
7	Glanders	Shirō Ishii, Tachiomaru Ishikawa
8	Tetanus	Shirō Ishii and more
9	Anaerobes	Unrecorded
10	B Hystolyticus	Unrecorded
11	B Welchii	Unrecorded
12	B Vovgii	Unrecorded
13	Undulant fever	Shirō Ishii, Yujiro Yamauchi, Kozo Yamamoto , Kiyoshi Hayakawa
14	Tuberculosis	Hideo Futatsugi, Shirō Ishii
15	Tularaemia	Shirō Ishii
16	Typhus	Shiro Kasahara, Den Masayoshi, Masaji Kitano, Tachiomaru Ishikawa
17	Songo	Shiro Kasahara, Masaji Kitano, Tachiomaru Ishikawa
18	Gas Gangrene	Shirō Ishii
19	Smallpox	Shirō Ishii, Tachiomaru Ishikawa
20	Aerosols	Masahiro Takahashi, Junichi Kaneko
21	Botulism	Shirō Ishii
22	Fugu Toxin	Tomohisa Masuda
23	Influenza	Shirō Ishii
24	Meningococcus	Shirō Ishii, Tachiomaru Ishikawa
25	Mucin	Ueda Masaaki, Uchino Snji
26	Plant Disease	Yukimasa Yagisawa

27	Salmonella	Kiyoshi Hayakawa, Seiwa Tanabe, Saburo Kojima
28	Tick encephalitis	Shiro Kasahara, Masaji Kitano
29	Tsutsugamushi	Shiro Kasahara

Production of Bacterial Agents

Unit 731 established divisions of bacterial research and experimentation to produce the bacterial agents of plague and cholera. Bacterial agents were the essential element. Unit 731 was concerned with keeping costs low and with producing powerful toxins with strong resistance to external forces and low traceability. Its staff utilised the latest technology and facilities to produce such agents.

From research and production to storage and transportation, the system was closely supervised. It conducted research on methods of attack with bacteriological warfare including hand-thrown or gun-delivered bombs, spray, aerial bombs, and bacteria-infected modes of delivery.

During the trial in Khabarovsk, the head of the Unit 731 bacteria production division, Kawashima Kiyoshi, claimed: 'Unit 731 could produce 800 to 900 kilograms of salmonella typhoid, 600 kilograms of anthrax, 1000 kilograms of cholera, paratyphoid and dysentery each month.'[6] As to quantity of production, Kawashima continued: '… the following are the amounts produced in one month: 100 kilograms of Yersinia pastis, anthrax 200 kilograms, 300 kilograms typhoid bacteria, 300 kilograms paratyphoid A, 330 kilograms cholera and 300 kilograms dysentery bacteria.'[7]

In 1942, during bacteriological warfare in Zhejiang-Jiangxi, Kawashima's division produced 130 kilograms of typhoid and anthrax for use in war.[8] In addition to Unit 731, other bacteria production divisions were involved in production and research, including Changchun Unit 100, Beijing Unit 1855, Nanjing Unit 1644, and Guangzhou Unit 860. Vast quantities of bacterial agents were produced by Unit 731 alone, and if the entire amount was used, there would be another worldwide disaster similar to the Black Death in Europe during the fourteenth century.

Battles of Khalkhin Gol

From May to September 1939, battles at the Soviet–Japanese border took place involving Japan, Manchukou, the Soviet Union, and Mongolia. Japan eventually lost. According to the Japanese National Archive, at 12 p.m. on 7 July 1939, Kanto Army Command Number 78, Kanto Army commander Ueda Kenkichi, issued commands to Army Surgeon Colonel Shirō Ishii: '… must depart for General Temple at Hailar District on July 8 and give assistance to the epidemic prevention and water supply division there. In order to bring facilities and supplies, 50 [men] of officer rank or below are allow to go along. It is necessary to report all the names who go with you' (see Fig. 30).[9]

Unit 731 launched the first bacteriological warfare at the direction of the Kanto Army. With the assistance of the Kanto Army, Lt-Col. Kichiro Yamamoto and

Tsuneshige Ikari of Unit 731 put cholera, typhoid fever, and shigella into the water supplies, including the Halha River. Yoshitaka Tamura of Unit 731 stated:

> ... under the command of technician Yamaguchi of the Kanto Army epidemic prevention and water supply division, around six members produced bacteria-[treated] shrapnel and about 2000 bullets. Members of Yamaguchi division shot the bacteria bombs in front of Khalkhin Gol. From early July to late August 1939, I joined the bacteria production division at Kobayashi, which was responsible for producing typhoid, cholera and epidemic typhus bacteria. I transported 1000 grams of bacteria to General Temple, Hailar District. I and the other three members from Tabei division put 1ml of bacterial liquid [which included 30 mg of typhoid] into two kerosene barrels. The next day I and the other two members brought the two barrels to General Temple and handed them to warrant officer Namba of the Kanto Army epidemic prevention and water supply division. Those bacterial agents that I brought were all spread into Halha River and started the bacteriological warfare.[10] [See Figures 31, 32, and 33.]

Unit 731 launched at least four bacteriological attacks in the battles of Khalkhin Gol. The preceding photographs from the National Institute for Defense Studies capture the work of Unit 731 in those battles. Since water was polluted by bacterial agents, Unit 731 carried out large-scale water filtration to prevent Japanese soldiers being infected. The contribution of Shirō Ishii to Khalkhin Gol earned him a medal from Kanto Army headquarters.

Changde Bacteriological Warfare

On 4 November 1941, Japanese planes flew over Hunan Changde and dropped fleas, fringe, wheat, cotton, paper, and other things. The chief targets were Guandi Temple Street, Poultry Lane, and East Gate in Changde. On 11 November, the first case of plague infection was found. The victim was an eleven-year-old girl, Cai Taoer, who lived on Guandi Temple Street; Cai died on 13 November. More cases of plague infection and death were found in Changde. Chen Wengui, director of the health officer training team, went to Changde to investigate the case, and his 'Report on Plague in Hunan Changde' noted the extent, harm, and effects of plague.

Chen's report stated:

> Since November 11, seven days after the attack by the Japanese Army, plague was widespread in Changde. All reports from Papanicolaou tests were checked by Dr Chan Wengui and Dr Tan Xuehua. From the medical record, dissection and bacteria check, victims were plague infected. There were six cases of plague infected, and until November 24, a total of seventeen individuals died in the spread of plague.[11]

'The Xiangxi Plague Prevention Report' by Rong Qirong, former chairperson in the Central Department of Health and Epidemic Prevention Department of Republic of China, claimed: 'Between November 11, 1941 and July 9, 1942, there were total 42 plague infected victims in Changde and 37 of them died'. Due to lack of sanitation facilities in Changde, epidemic prevention was seriously delayed. People in Changde did not cooperate well, which led to the failure of plague prevention and inaccurate official data. The numbers in reports by Chen Wengui and Rong Qirong were too low. After the initial outbreak of plague in 1941, there were still fatalities as late as 1945. Chen's and Rong's reports recorded the spread of plague, which was attributed to fleas and plague-infected material dropped by Japanese planes. The outbreak of plague occurred seven days following the large-scale aerial bombardment. According to the investigation by Chen and Rong, the outbreak was due to this attack by the Japanese Army.

In November 1996, the Investigation Organisation of Bacteriological Warfare Victims was established in Changde. The civil organisation was formed by retired teachers, doctors, workers, and victims' families. According to statistics provided by the organisation from 1996 to 2002, more than 300,000 individuals from nine areas in Changde were interviewed. About 15,000 statements of accusation were collected. A total of 7,643 individuals from more than seventy towns and 486 villages died of plague. The investigation organisation published 'Name List of Victims and Surviving Dependents' that recorded the name, gender, and time and place of deaths in detail.

One case among the oral narratives from family members of victims had a deep impact on me. The case of Fang Yunsheng was written by Liu Yi from Hunan University of Arts and Science in '12 Cases of Oral Historical Research of Victims in Changde Bacteriological Warfare':

> ... my elder brother Fang Yundeng died in the 1941 plague in Changde. He died at age 8. After my brother died, my grandmother was very depressed and suffered a mental breakdown. She often walked along the streets and shouted my brother's name. She hoped my brother would come home. When I was a kid, my grandmother held my hand and shouted my brother's name on the street...[12]

Quzhou Bacteriological Warfare

According to the narrative of Mingxuan Qiu, former supervisor in the health and epidemic prevention station in Quzhou:

> ... at 9 o'clock on October 4, 1940, Japanese planes spread plague-infected fleas, wheat, soybeans, wheat bran, cloth, cotton and flyers. The plane flew back and forth twice and left Quzhou at around half past 9. In early December, the first plague happened in the history of Quzhou, and it spread all over the village area. On May 26, 1942, the Japanese army launched the second attack of bacteriological warfare in

Quzhou. The Japanese [used planes to] spread plague-inflected fleas, sent expedition troops to transportation lines between Zhe and Gan to spread fleas, as well as put cholera, typhoid and paratyphoid, dysentery and anthrax in the wells and on food of the civilians.[13]

In early September, sites along the transportation line between Zhe and Gan, such as Jiangshan, Quzhou, Kaihua, and Longyou, suffered outbreaks of plague, cholera, typhoid, paratyphoid, dysentery, malaria, and anthrax. At the same time, the Japanese Army began indiscriminate bombing of Quzhou, which worsened the work of epidemic prevention. Not until 1948 were the diseases thoroughly suppressed.

From 1998 to 2000, a few investigations were carried out in Quzhou. Aspects widely studied included source of infection, the spread of bacteria, and infected victims.

According to an investigative report about Quzhou, 5,294 people were victims of Japanese bacteriological warfare: 1,501 of plague, 909 of cholera, 2,272 of typhoid, 407 of dysentery, and 205 of anthrax; 3,748 were male and 1,546 were female; and 871 were children less than ten years old. The oldest victim was eighty-three and the youngest was three months. A large number of pregnant women died with their unborn babies.

In addition to causing large-scale plague in the Quzhou area, the Japanese Army launched bacteriological warfare in Jinhua, Yiwu, Ningbo, and Lishui in October 1940. According to the investigative report 'Name List of Victims in Bacteriological Warfare in Yiwu, Zhejiang (1941–1943)', 1,315 people there died due to Japanese bacteriological warfare.

Yunhe Zhejiang's 'Name List of Victims in Bacteriological Warfare in WWII' records 781 fatalities of Japanese bacteriological warfare. Based on the previous information, 15,033 victims died in bacteriological warfare in Changde, Yiwu, Yunhe, and Quzhou. Additional infected areas were left uninvestigated. The number of Chinese civilians, including women and children, is believed to be much higher than the number in the records.

Biochemical weapons were abandoned by the Japanese in more than 100 areas among nineteen provinces in China. The harmful effects of such weapons remain a threat to Chinese civilians. The largest number to date were found in Dunhua city in Jilin province, where 747 civilians died due to exposure to biochemical weapons. In 1974, three individuals were seriously harmed by abandoned biochemical weapons in Jiamusi city of Heilongjiang province. In 2003, in Qiqihaer in Heilongjiang province, leftover bacterial liquid killed one civilian and injured forty-three more.

According to informal records, since the end of the war, abandoned biochemical weapons have killed more than 2,000 civilians and caused widespread harm to property, the climate, and ecosystems. In 1995, Chinese civilians organised the Litigation Campaign for Chinese Victims Suffering from Japanese Poison Gases in Bacteriological Warfare. In Tokyo District Court on 15 May 2003, facing the evidence of numerous oral narratives, the Japanese had to admit that 'During war against China, the Japanese Army produced and used abundant amounts of biological weapons'.

The Japanese claimed that 'the Japanese government did not have effective means to prevent harm from happening', so the Chinese desire for an official apology and compensation from the Japanese government failed. The grassroots campaign was not supported or funded by the Chinese government, which made it difficult to sustain without the backing of organised authority. Questions persist: victims went to the abuser's country to litigate on behalf of their country with assistance from attorneys of the abuser's country. What is the percentage of success under these circumstances? What is the future of the litigation?

The Harm of War: Spread of Plague in Pingfang

In preparing and launching bacteriological warfare, Unit 731 purchased a large number of animals for experimental use. Due to the length of time, scale, and number of species, domestic animal life systems and ecosystems were widely violated. Plague and other bacteria turned the Pingfang area into living 'gunpowder barrels'. When Unit 731 escaped from Harbin after the end of the Second World War, and although the Japanese bombed most of the facilities and animals, a number of mice, fleas, and other experimental animals fled the cages. The exploration of 'bacterial gunpowder barrels' led to the wide outbreak of plague in Pingfang.

In July 1946, Dong Xu, wife of Hongyou Xu, from Erdaogou of Pingfang area was the first to die of plague. Later, Ruxian Jing was infected by plague, and his wife, Song Jing, and their children, ages five and two, died of plague. Seven of nineteen members of the Jing family died within twenty days. Jing's son Jing Fuhe recalled the disaster:

My home in Pingfang area was the severely affected area. Within no more than 20 days, 12 out of 19 members of my family were killed by plague. When my father, older sister and younger brother fell down, the other family members were also infected. Those who were alive could not take care of them much, and they got infected eventually. My mother was taking care of my father, and I was with my younger brother. My father and my younger brother stayed in the same bed and there was no space for my sister. So we put her on the grass, like she was waiting for death. My older sister's symptom was a low fever. There were bumps on her neck and swellings. She could not speak. She lay on the grass, no one stayed by her side, and she died alone screaming. The hearse had not yet arrived wen my father died as well. Before we took his body out of the bed, my younger brother spat black saliva twice. He died with his eyes open. I was with my younger brother. I yelled his name and tried to talk to him, but he never replied. I watched my younger brother lose his life. Whenever I think of the disaster, I cry and I feel extremely sad. The screams of my father, the way my older sister died alone, and my younger brother wide open eyes, I can never forget.[14] [See Fig. 34.]

In total, fifty people died from plague in Erdaogou. The youngest was two years old and the oldest was seventy-one. In some families, all members perished. Plague outbreaks also took place in Yifayuantun (forty-one cases) and Dongjingzi (thirty-eight cases) at the same time.

According to the 'Report on Plague Prevention in Harbin' maintained by the Heilongjiang Provincial Archive in 1946, there were no basic epidemic prevention facilities, doctors, or clinics in villages in Pingfang. The city of Harbin started epidemic prevention, isolation, disinfection, and vaccination two months after the plague outbreak, and by 1945, the plague was finally under control.

Although Unit 731 disbanded in 1945, the harm to Harbin did not vanish along with it. From 1946 to 1954, 143 people died of plague. The Chinese of Harbin suffered heavy mental pressure and serious economic harm, and the violated ecosystem and the change in conditions of mice continued to cause plague in Harbin area. Post-war Pingfang became the world's sole centre suffering from human-caused plague.

From 1954 to 1994, the city of Harbin applied human resources, facilities, and financial support to improve protection against plague. Finally, in 1994, according to the report on plague monitoring issued by the epidemic protection station in Harbin, 'the result of plague testing of mice in Harbin is negative, which means the outbreak of plague in Harbin is finally under control after 49 years'.

Investigation, Cover-up, and Exchange

With the surrender of Japan announced by Emperor Hirohito, the Second World War came to an official end on 15 August 1945. US President Harry S. Truman appointed Gen. Douglas MacArthur as Supreme Commander for the Allied Powers, and MacArthur accepted the surrender of Emperor Hirohito aboard the USS *Missouri*.

During this period, before the start of the Cold War and the spread of Communist ideology, in order to control post-war Japan under the US's choice of ideological and political systems, the US took the lead in the International Military Tribunal for the Far East (also known as the Tokyo Trials) slated to try Japanese war criminals. Beginning in September 1945, the US Army initiated investigation into Japanese biological warfare. The investigation ended November 1948. Over four years, the US Army successfully enacted a secret agreement with the Japanese government allowing members of Unit 731 to avoid trial.

At the end of the Second World War, members of Unit 731, including Shirō Ishii and Masaji Kitano, returned to Japan where many of them lived secretly, changed their names, or faked their deaths to escape trial. The US Army sought statistics and data on Japanese biological warfare and experiments carried out by Unit 731, therefore, prior to the Tokyo Trials, the US intelligence agency investigated Ishii, Kitano, and other members of the unit. At least twenty-five members were tried by the US Army; however, Ishii and others were exempted from trial.

Tracking Shirō Ishii

The US Intelligence Agency paid primary attention to the founder of Unit 731, Shirō Ishii, rating him the most wanted person by the US authorities. The Second Division of the General Staff Headquarters in Tokyo had assigned intelligence agents to track him down for a long time.

Fraudulent Death of Shirō Ishii

Three months before the Tokyo Trials, Ishii faked his death to evade trial, but twenty days later, the US Intelligence Agency uncovered his deception. According to the information collected from the Intelligence Agency: '... on December 3, 1945, an informer of the US Army reported that Shirō Ishii had arranged a fake funeral for himself at his hometown Chiyoda village at Sanbugun, Chiba on November 10, 1945. He, however, remained hidden with the help of the head villager. Shirō Ishii was the Lieutenant General and head of Ishii Division and was in charge of human experimentation during the war'.[1]

More information on Ishii was contained in a US Army memo dated 3 December:

The biological warfare division was established in Harbin under the command of Shirō Ishii. In December 1944, a large-scale bacteria laboratory had successfully cultured Yersinia pastis in Harbin. This bacteria was released throughout Manchuria. In Shenyang, some US POWs were injected with *Yersinia pestis*. In order to observe the experiment results, the biological warfare division released infected mice in Shenyang and other areas to create large-scale plague. After these experiments, Shirō Ishii noted the need to culture *Yersinia pestis* for use in warfare. When Japan was defeated, the Japanese Army destroyed laboratories as well as abundant important information, facilities and hundreds of '*marutas*' [prisoners]. Ishii's biological warfare division had cooperated with the Department of Medicine in the University of Tokyo.[2]

The US Army documented Ishii's activities, especially his involvement in the Harbin laboratory, human experimentation, and biological warfare, as well as his collaboration with the University of Tokyo. This information had reached the core of Unit 731— human experimentation and biological warfare.

Information from the Intelligence Agency: Discovery of Shirō Ishii

A US Army record, dated 28 December 1945, states: 'Shirō Ishii left Harbin with about $1 million cash. Shirō Ishii was suspected by the Intelligence Agency for not being arrested as war criminal'.[3] Another US Army record, dated 7 January 1946, states:

According to comment from the United States Department of Defense made on January 6, 1946, Shirō Ishii committed biological experiments in Manchuria and should be arrested and interrogated. The record from the Secret Intelligence Service and military could not reveal the location of Shirō Ishii, and it did not request the Japanese government to arrest Shirō Ishii for the US Army.[4]

On 7 January 1946, members of the US Intelligence Agency interviewed Ralph Teatsorth and S. E. Whitesides of the United Forces Association in the Tokyo

Broadcasting Building. Teatsorth provided information on 'Shirō Ishii's involvement in plague injection of American and Chinese POWs', and Whitesides presented proof of Ishii's involvement in biological warfare and the Unit 731 Bacteria Division.[5] Neither man knew Ishii's location. Four days after the release of Teatsorth's information, on 11 January, he interrogated the second in command of Unit 731, Masaji Kitano, who provided further information about biological experiments and bacteria bombs. The US Intelligence Agency put great effort into tracing Shirō Ishii in order to collect details on human experimentation, which made Ishii the man most wanted by the Agency.

On 8 January 1946, an informant provided clues about Shirō Ishii's location: 'Shirō Ishii went to the Kanazawa area. Professor Tachio Ishikawa (石川太刀雄) from the Department of Pathology in Kanazawa University knew Ishii's location'.[6]

The following day, the US Army received information from the Central Liaison Office in Tokyo: 'The Japan Imperial Government would like to turn over Shirō Ishii to Tokyo for interrogation by the Supreme Commander for the Allied Powers. When Shirō Ishii arrived in Tokyo, the Imperial Government would contact the Allied Powers as soon as possible. If Ishii did not arrive by midnight January 16, 1946, the Imperial Government would provide a detailed report explaining Ishii's location and reason for his absence in order to suggest his arrival date'.[7]

At that time, neither the US Army nor Japanese official agencies officially knew Ishii's whereabouts, but the possibility of the Japanese government's intentional cover-up should not be ignored.

The US Army stated its intentions back on 2 January 1946: 'The Secret Intelligence Service and military requested information related to biological warfare and wished to collect further valuable information'.[8] Yet weeks had passed with no results as the prime target remained in hiding.

On 19 January 1946, the International Military Tribunal for the Far East was established and announced its charter. The Tokyo Trials were about to start, and the deadline of 16 January, as set by the Japanese government, had passed. The Tokyo Central Office contacted Professor Tachio Ishikawa regarding Ishii's location without results. The Intelligence Agency suggested that the Tokyo Central Office failed to provide the location of Shirō Ishii and his arrival date in Tokyo.

Appearance of Ishii

The US Army found Shirō Ishii on 5 February 1946, and A. T. Thompson began his interrogation.

On 16 February, the Secret Intelligence Service and military sent Civil Intelligence Section a list of those connected to Shirō Ishii, including Kanji Ishiwara, Masaji Kitano, Ryoichi Naito, Enryo Houjyo, Nishimura Eiji, Hisato Yoshimura, and nineteen others. The ongoing interrogation was recorded; however, there was, as yet, no substantiation of the use of living humans in experimentation.

According to US Army records of 11 March 1946: 'Shirō Ishii needed to report his address to the US Army when he returned home to Chiba prefecture. The Intelligence Agency planned to interrogate Ishii, and he needed to be ready for interrogation at any time'.[9]

According to US Army records of 16 March: 'Shirō Ishii did not report to the US Army. He made up an excuse of illness to stay in Tokyo. Shirō Ishii's wife, Ishii Kiyoko, said Shirō Ishii would go back to Chiba prefecture and report to the US Army when he arrived'.[10]

The US Army record of 1 April states: 'Shirō Ishii did not report his address in Chiba prefecture to the US Army.[11] Six months after the surrender of Japan, the US Army had found Shirō Ishii and Masaji Kitano, a breakthrough in uncovering the secrets of Unit 731, human experimentation, and biological warfare.

Secret Investigation and Interrogation by the US Army

The US Department of Defense led the investigation into Japanese biological warfare. With the assistance of the Supreme Commander for the Allied Powers, the US Army carried out a series of secret investigations from the end of the Second World War through late 1948. Murray Sanders, A. T. Thompson, Norbert Fell, and Edwin V. Hill from the Fort Detrick, Maryland, military base wrote concluding reports regarding their investigations of the Japanese officers.

Investigation by Murray Sanders

Prior to the end of the war, the US Army had learned of biological warfare carried out by Japanese troops in Hunan and Zhejiang, China. After war's end, the US treated it as a highly confidential matter and tried every method to obtain access to documentation. Murray Sanders, a biological warfare expert from the Detrick military base, arrived in Japan soon after the surrender and conducted an investigation from September to October 1945. Sanders interrogated the Japanese Army Hospital School, Imperial Japanese Army General Staff Office, members of the Ministry of War of Japan and important members including Ryoichi Naito, Junichi Kaneko, and Tomohisa Masuda. Unfortunately, Sanders failed to find the escapee, Shirō Ishii. On 1 November 1946, Sanders completed his 'Japanese Intelligence Information Investigation Report—Biological Warfare', often known as 'The Sanders Report'.

'The Sanders Report' covered research areas, operation system, duties, Unit 731 members, organisations, production records of vaccines, and bacteria. A map of Pingfang area and design plans of bacteria bombs were included. Sanders received important information about the core mission of Unit 731 from the Japanese interviewees that the Japanese had made tremendous efforts to develop the biological experiments into practical weapons, at least eight kinds of special bombs able to disperse large quantities of bacteria were tested experimentally. The most advanced weapon was the UJ150 bomb, of which over 2,000 were tested. The tests were carried out by static blasting and air bombing in the Pingfang area, using more than 4,000 bombs.[12] The report recorded details of the experiment, statistics, the model number of bombs, and field human experimentation. These details assisted the US Army investigation of biological warfare, human experimentation, and biological weapons of Unit 731.

Investigation by A. T. Thompson

Col. A. T. Thompson, a biological warfare expert from the Detrick base, arrived in Japan to investigate Unit 731 after Sanders departed. A military veterinarian, Col. Thompson interrogated members of Unit 731, including Ishii and Kitano, and members of Unit 100 (Thompson committed suicide in 1948 for unknown reasons).

First Meeting with Investigator
On 5 February 1946, Thompson visited the home of Shirō Ishii. The interrogation began and ended in a cordial atmosphere. The following narrative is an excerpt of the report:

Q: You did no BW work except at the Army Medical College and at Heibo?

A: BW work was done only at Heibo. Only general preventive medical science was conducted at the Army Medical College.

Q: Was any work done at the Kyoto Imperial University?

A: The professor there did not like that kind of work, so none was undertaken.

Q: The research work was limited to Heibo institute?

A: Only at Heibo. A lot of men in my unit and others who do not know anything about it have been spreading rumours to the effect that some secret work has been carried on in BW and they have gone as far as saying an attack with BW was planned by my unit and that a lot of bacteria were being produced, large quantities of bombs manufactured and airplanes being gathered for that purpose. I want you to have a clear understanding that this is false.

Q: In other words, no work was conducted on BW except at the Heibo institute?

A: That is correct

Q: Did you except the enemy to use BW?

A: In my opinion, some countries might.

Q: Which countries did you expect to use it?

A: Soviet Union and China. They had used it previously and I expected them to use it again.

Q: What did expect from the United States in the field of BW?

A: I did not think the United States would use BW.

Q: Why?

A: I believed since the United States had money and materials, they would use more scientific method of warfare.

Q: Do you think BW is practical?

A: You have to have much money and materials to create conditions favourable to BW.

Q: Do you think BW is something that nations will have to contend with in the future?

A: In a winning war, there is no necessity for using BW and in a losing war, there is not the opportunity to use BW effectively. You need a lot of men, money and materials to conduct research into BW. There is little data on the effectiveness of BW as a weapon. I do not know whether BW can be used effectively on a large scale. It might be effective on a small scale.

Q: Do you mean sabotage?

A: It might be effective in such methods of sabotage as dropping bacteria into wells.

Q: It might be effective under those conditions?

A: I believe such methods could be controlled by my methods of water purification. I heard over the radio that Russia had completed its preparations for BW and it frightened me, but I did not know whether it was actual fact or just was printed in 'Red Star' or some other newspaper as a 'scare'. I do not know how far they have advanced in BW and have wondered what they would use if they attacked with BW.

Q: What bacteria do you think the Russians might use?

A: Tularaemia, typhus fever, cholera, anthrax, pest.

Q: What makes you believe that the Russians would use these organisms?

A: I heard reports from people returned from Russia that the Russians had been using these organisms in their preparation for BW.

Q: Would it not be difficult to produce typhus organisms on a large scale?

A: If you could produce a lot of lice you might be able to produce a lot of typhus. German and Polish vaccine is prepared from lice. Trouble with lice is that you have to have human infectious blood to infect the lice. Weil's disease is produced in the same manner and it is very hard to get large quantities. If a country was rich enough, it might be able to make that disease a dangerous weapon.

Q: Was any research conducted on BW against food plants?

A: We did not do any experiments on it. Our work was to protect the soldiers.

Q: Did anyone else concern themselves with BW against crop plants?

A: I do not know.

Q: Were you concerned with BW agents against animals?

A: We did not do any experiments on large animals. We used small animals as test animals. Besides, we had no veterinarians.

Q: Did veterinary laboratories do any research on BW?

A: I do not know. It was such a secret that there was no communication between units. Even personnel working on experiments in my unit did not know what they were working on. Only myself, Colonel MASUDA, and one or two other persons know.

Q: Who were the other persons?

A: There were some who suspected what was going on, but did not know. Colonel MASUDA, Tomosada, and myself know.

Q: What section of the BW institute did the BW work?

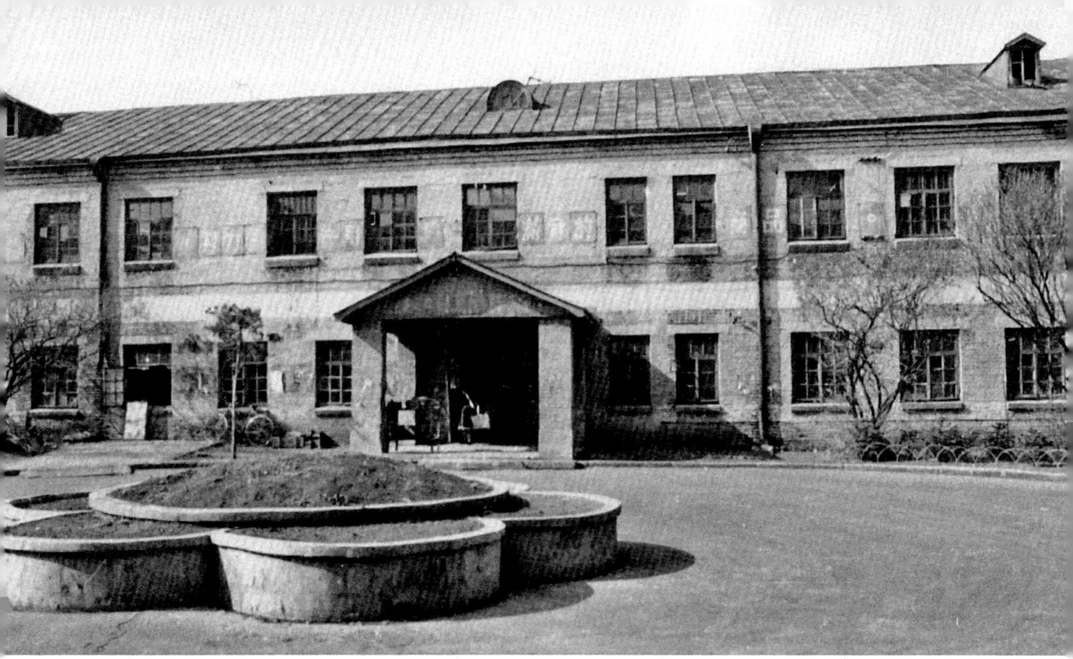

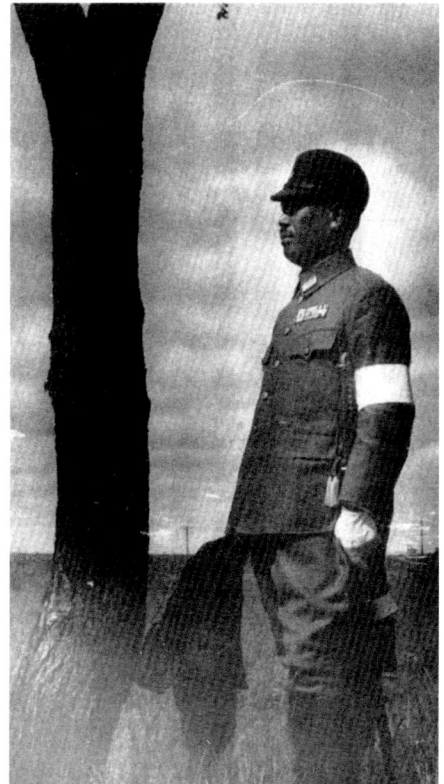

Above: Fig. 1 Early Unit 731.

Top right: Fig. 2 Employee's Card of Unit 731.

Centre right: Fig. 3 Labour Certification of Unit 731.

Bottom right: Fig. 4 Shirō Ishii.

Bottom left: Fig. 5 Masaji Kitano.

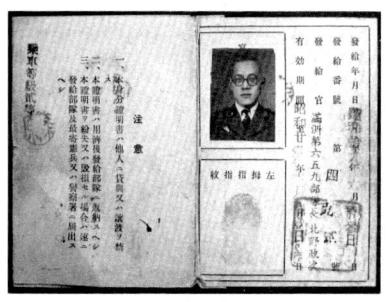

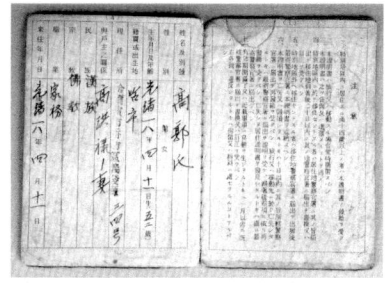

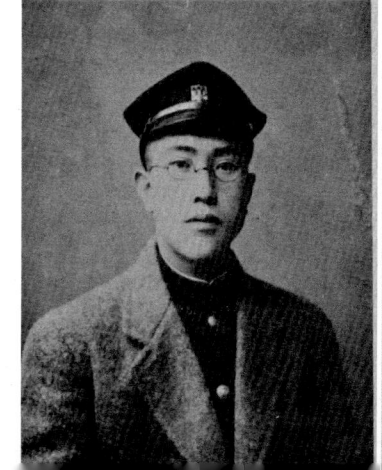

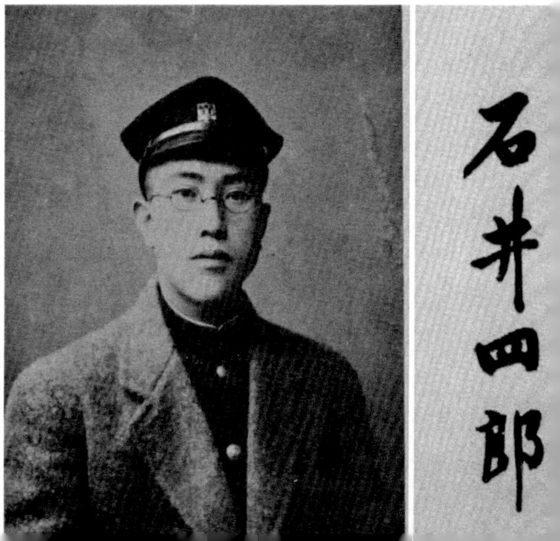

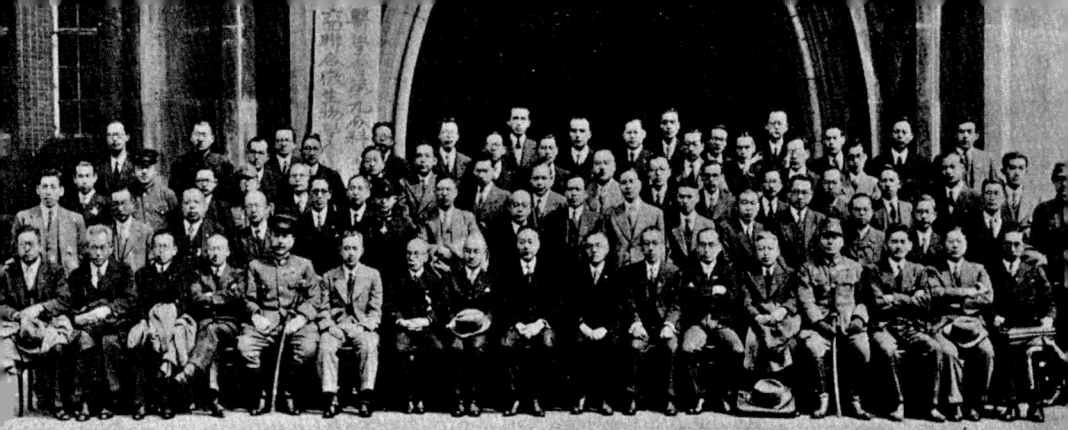

Fig. 6 The 11th Meeting of the Japanese Association of Medicinal Sciences. Shirō Ishii.

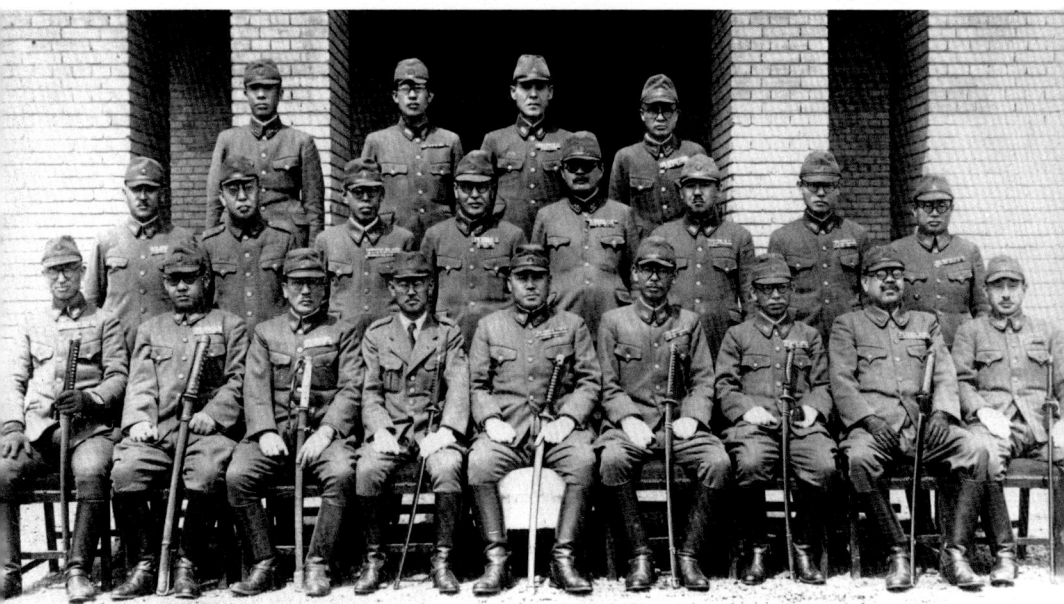

Fig. 7 The senior officers of Unit 731. Masaji Kitano (front row, in the middle).

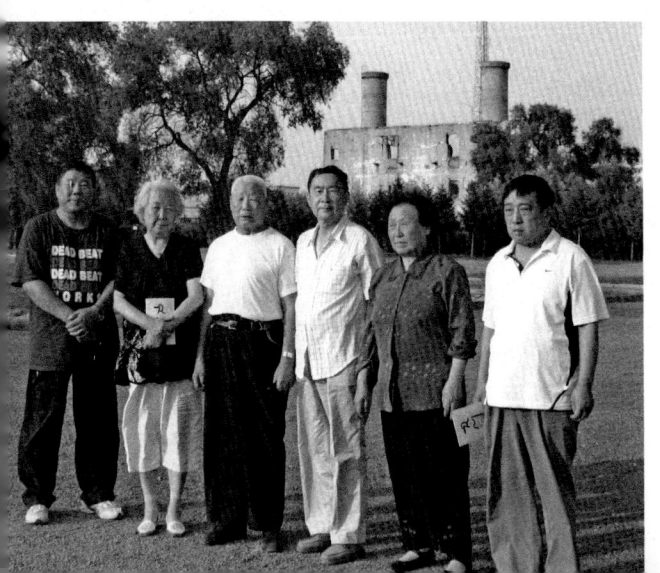

Left: Fig. 8 Victims' family members, taken at the former site of Unit 731. *From left to right*: Xiaoguang Wang, Fengqin Li, Yibang Wang, Kewei Zhang (son of victim Huizhong Zhang), Yufen Zhu (daughter of victim Yuntong Zhu), and the son of Yufen Zhu. (*Kept by International Center for Unit 731 Research*)

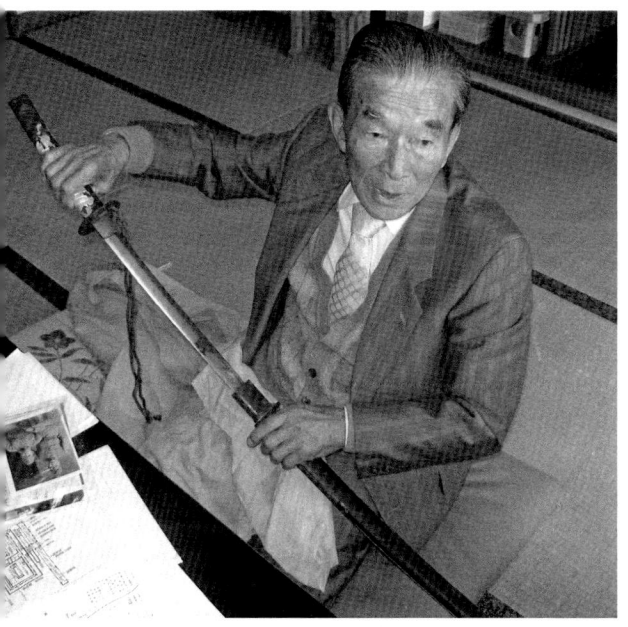
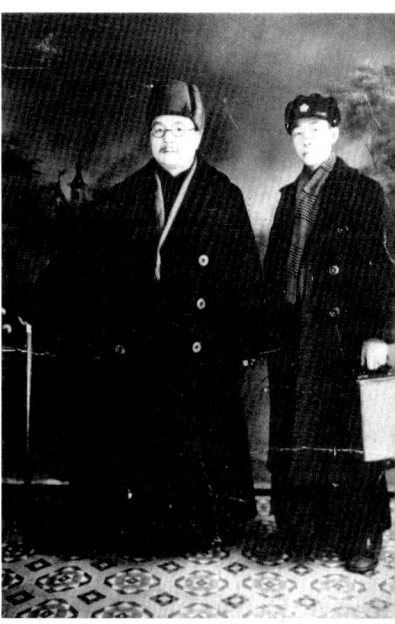

Above left: Fig. 9 Okawa Fukumatsu, 2008.

Above right: Fig. 10 Victims of Special Transfer: Yaoxuan Wang and Xuenian Wang.

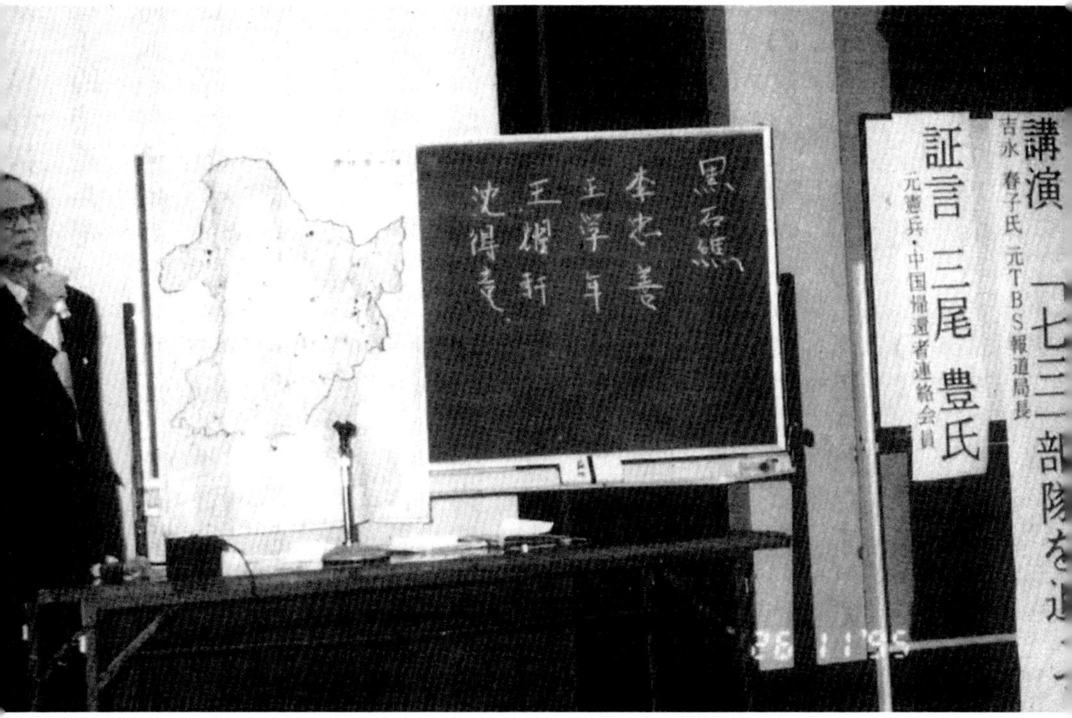

Fig. 11 On 26 November 1995, Yutaka Mio shared his oral narrative on Unit 731 Exhibition Tour in Japan. *Renzuizhilu: Qisanyibudui yu sanweifeng de jilu* (Trip of Crime Committing: Record of Unit 731 and Yutaka Mio).

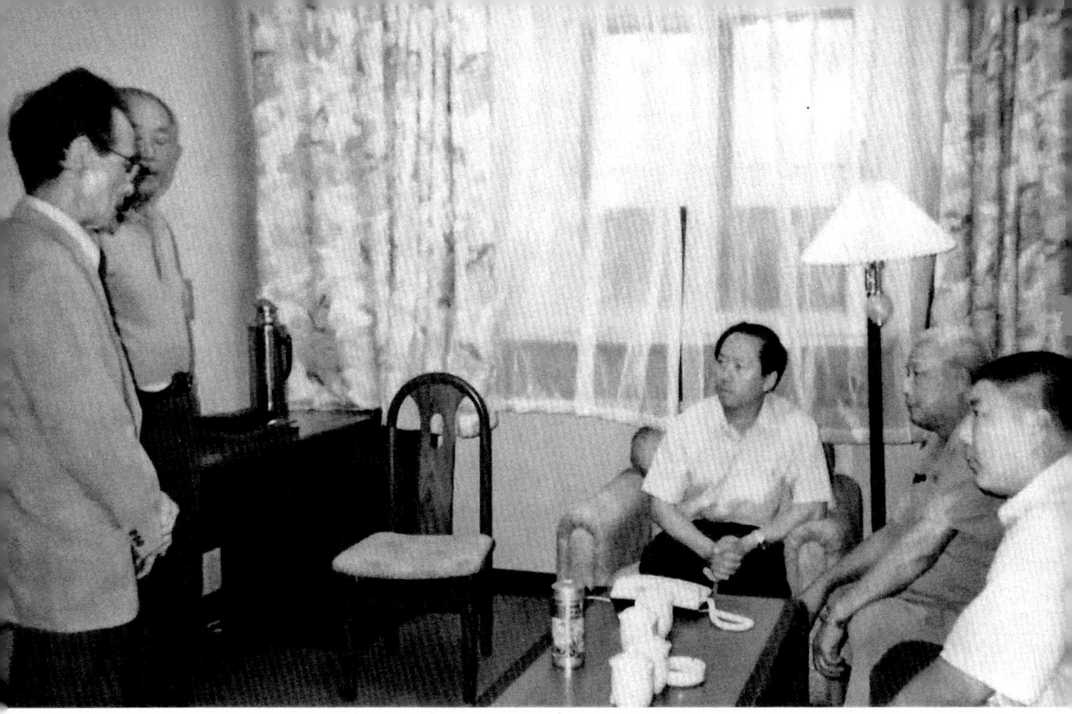

Above: Fig. 12 On 31 July 1995, Yutaka Mio apologised to Yibing Wang and Xiaoguang Wang. *From left to right*: Yutaka Mio, former director of Fushun War Criminals Management Centre Yuan Jin, Wenjun Shi from Dalian Chronicle Office, Yibing Wang (son of Yaoxuan Wang) and Xiaoguang Wang (grandson of Yaoxuan Wang). (*Photo provided by Yibing Wang*)

Below: Fig. 13 On 11 April 2015, author Yan-jun Yang (left) interviewed Yibing Wang. *From right to left*: Rujia Liu and Tongzhu Wang.

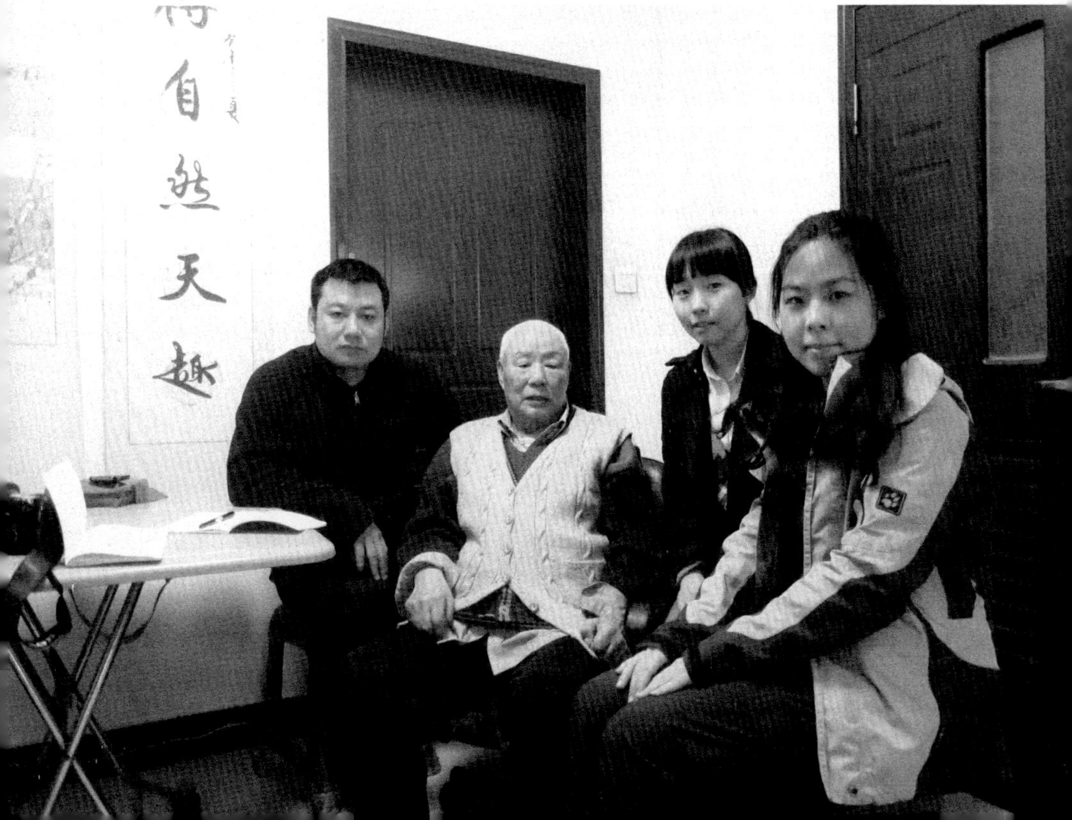

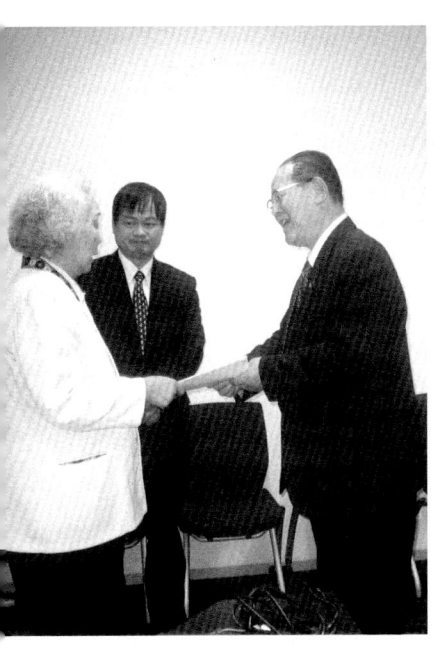

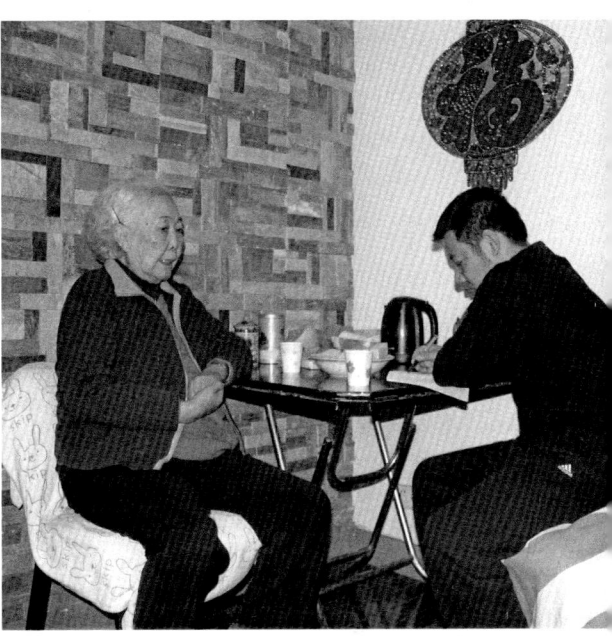

Above left: Fig. 14 On 24 November 2010, Fengqin Li handed the application to the Japan Parliamentarians' Union and discussed her father's history. (*Photo courtesy of International Center for Unit 731 Research*)

Above right: Fig. 15 On 12 April 2015, the author interviewed Fengqin Li. (*Photo by Tongzhu Wang*)

Below: Fig. 16 Pengge Li (first at left) and classmates at graduation. (*Photo provided by Fengqin Li*)

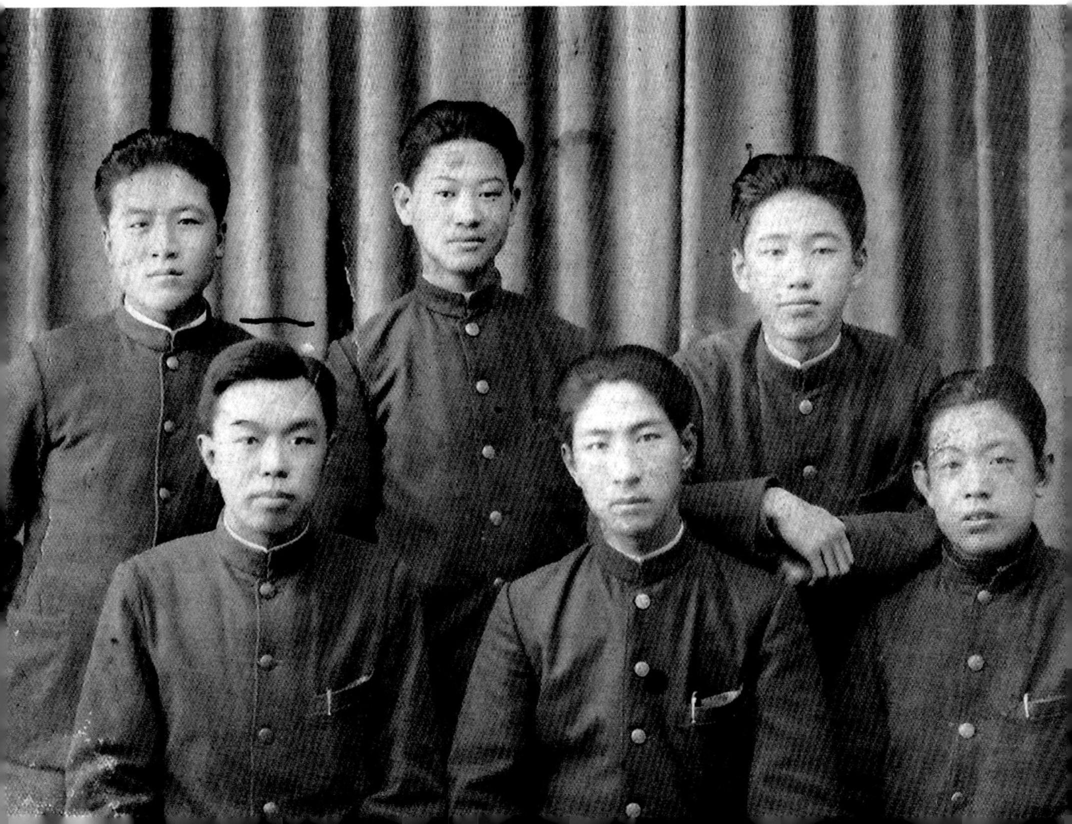

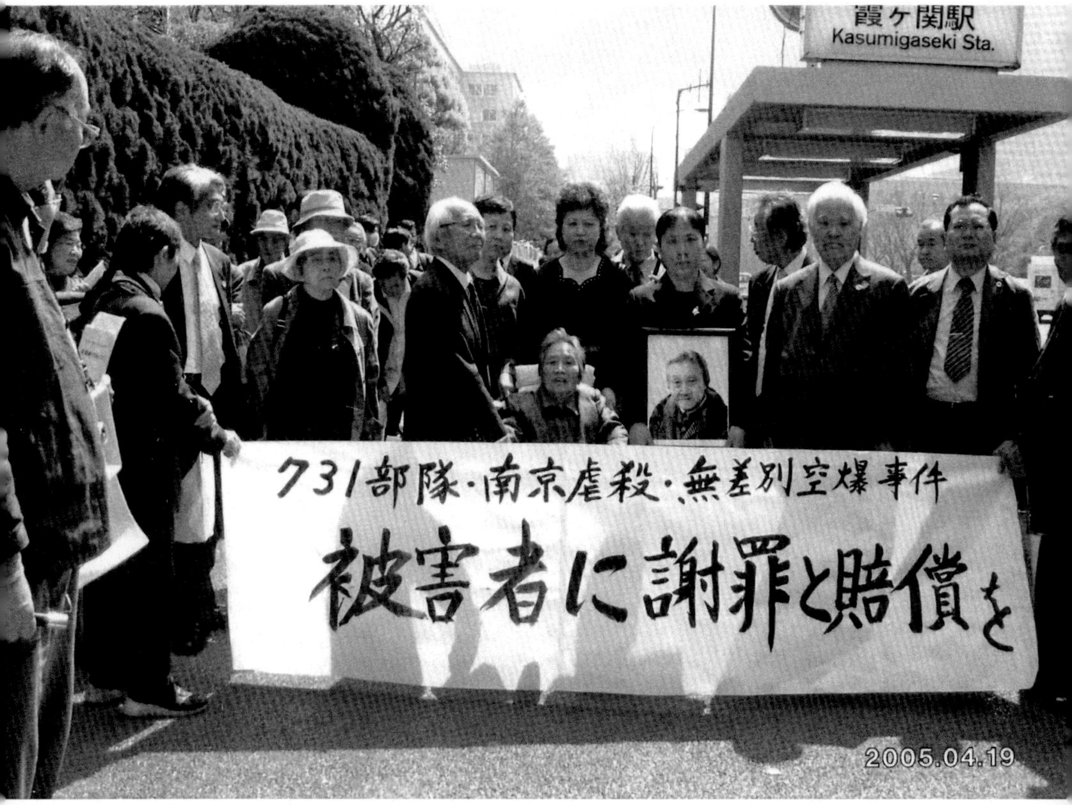

![Figure 17 photograph]

Fig. 17 On 18 April 2005, Lanzhi Jing (in wheelchair) visited Japan for an appeal. The man in glasses (standing at left next to Jing) is former Unit 731 member Yoshio Shinozuka. (*Photo provided by Japanese ABC Project Organisation*)

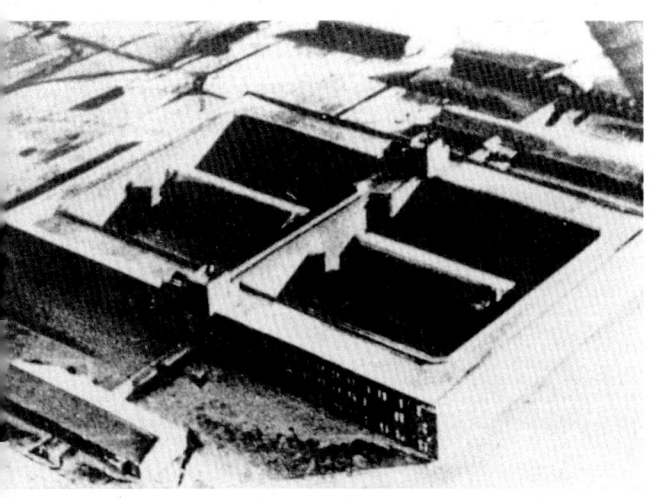

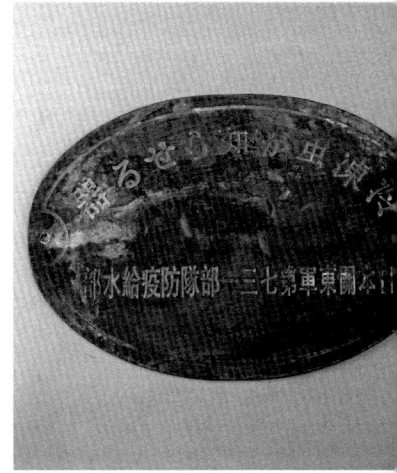

Above left: Fig. 18 Square Quarter of Unit 731. Taken by the aviation class and photography class of Unit 731 in August 1940. (*Kadokawa Bunko Press, 2008*).

Above right: Fig. 19 Cold anticipator. The caption reads: 'Epidemic Prevention and Water Purification Department of the Unit 731, Japan's Kwantung Army'. (*Photo provided by Zhang Guangsheng*)

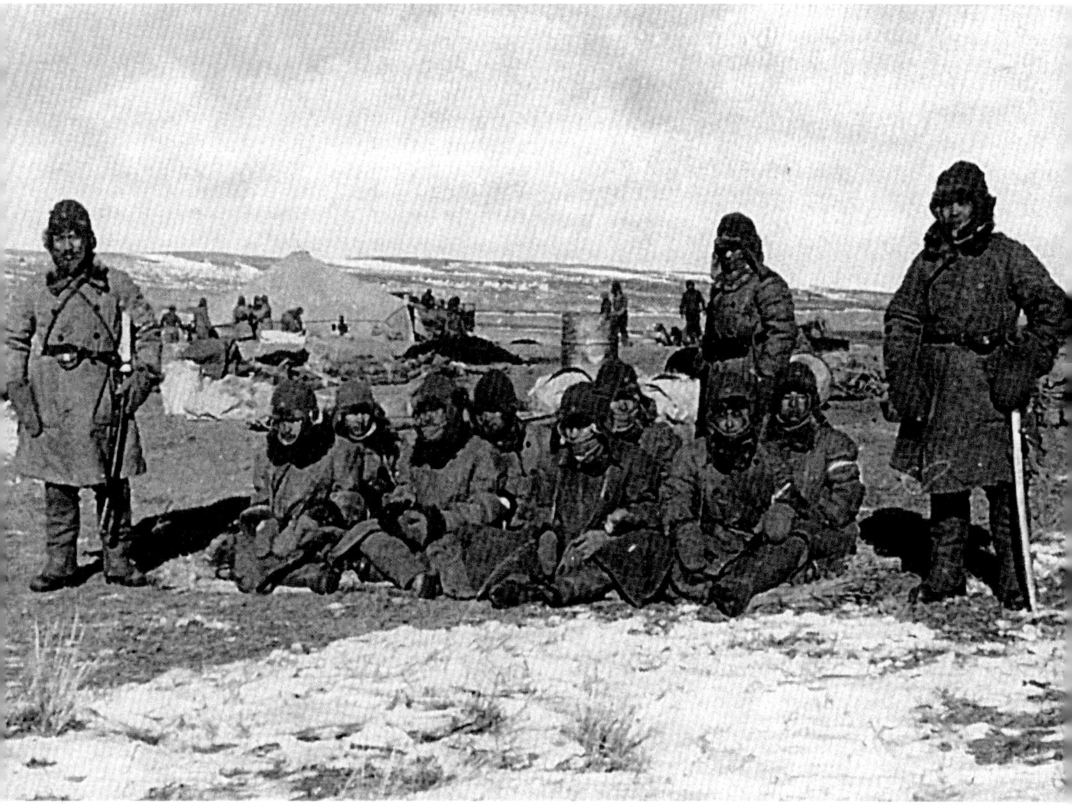

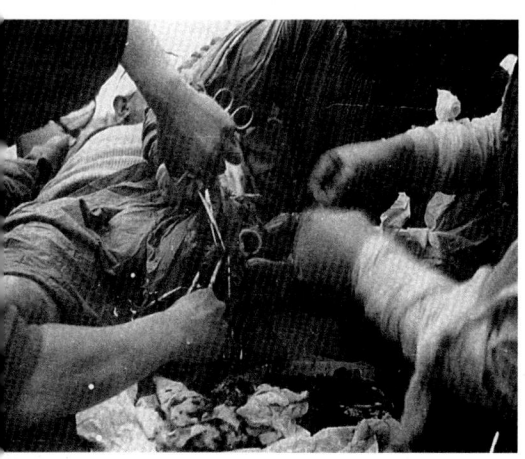

Fig, 20 Japanese soldiers monitor eight experimental subjects sitting on grassland before the frostbite experiment.

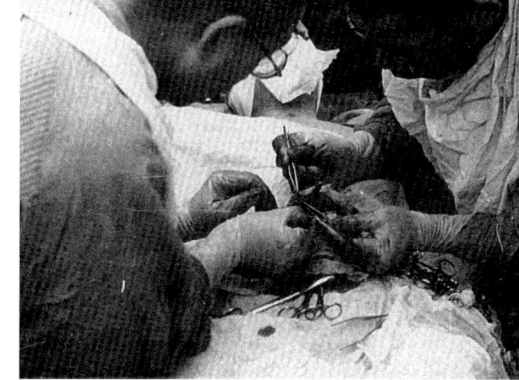

Fig. 21 Japanese soldiers conducting vivisection.

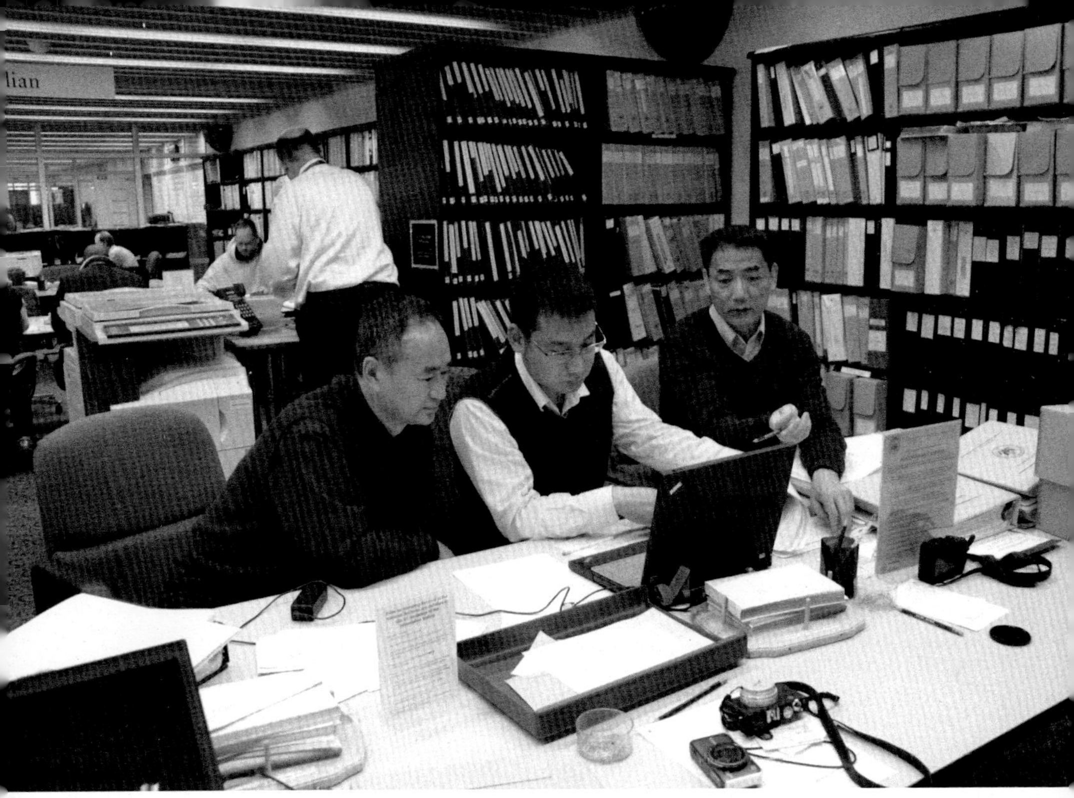

Above: Fig. 22 Author Yan-jun Yang (middle) researching at the National Archives and Records Administration II. Haichun Bao (left) and Yuwu Song (right). (*Photo by Liu Rujia*)

Below: Fig. 23 Mr Yan-jun Yang (left) received Report 'A' and Report 'G' at the Science, Technology and Business Division of the Library of Congress, US. Tomoko Y. Steen is at right. (*Photo by Bao Haichun*)

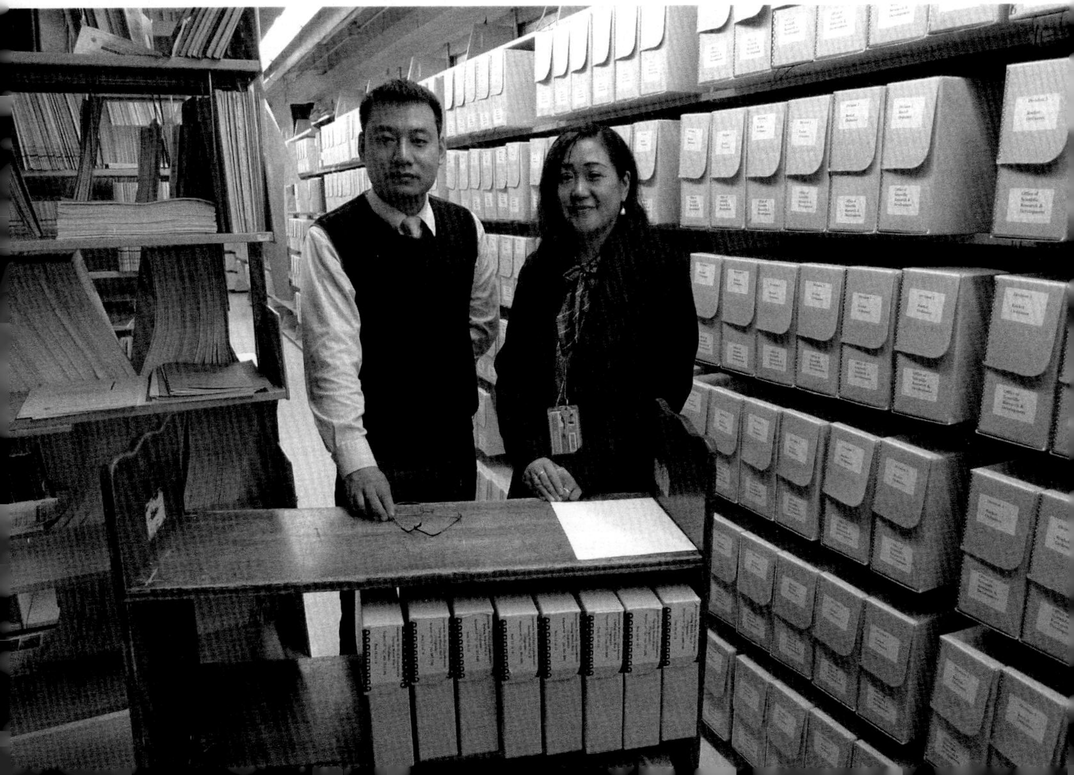

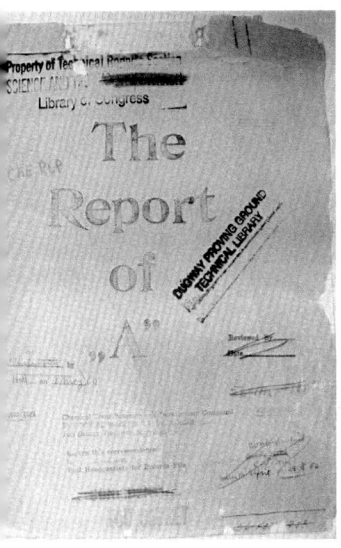
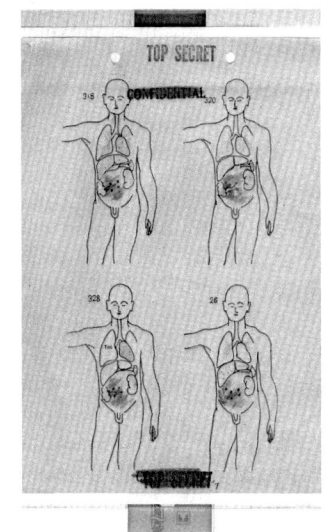
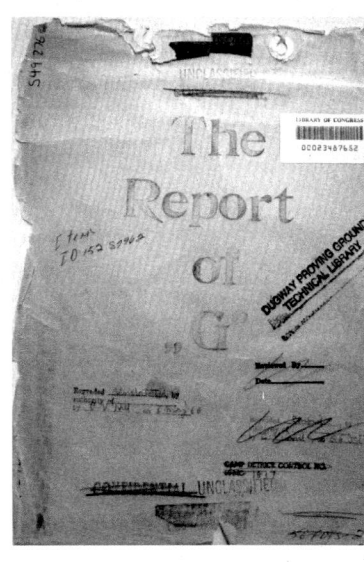

Above left: Fig. 24 Cover of Report 'A' on Human Experimentation by Anthrax. (*Library of Congress, US*)

Above middle: Fig. 25 Organ infection record in Report 'A'. (*Library of Congress, US*)

Above right: Fig. 26 Cover of Report 'G' on Human Experimentation by Glanders. (*Library of Congress, US*)

Below left: Fig. 27 Illustration of bacteria bombs Model 50, Model 100, Model GA, Older Model UJI, Model RO, Model I, Model U, and Model HA.

Below right: Fig. 28 'Thompson's Report'.

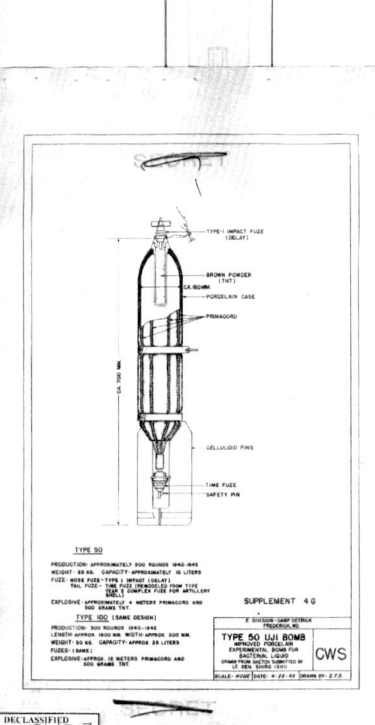
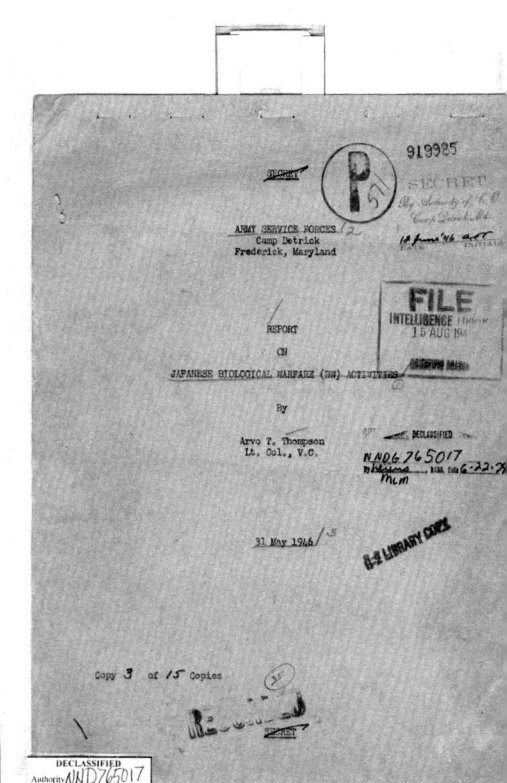

1246

極秘

關作命丙第七八號

關東軍命令 新京

陸軍軍醫大佐 石井四郎

七月八日ヨリ十日間ノ豫定ヲ以テ
海拉爾、將軍廟方面ニ到リ防疫給
水部隊ノ指導ニ任スヘシ
器材補給ノ爲部下將校以下十五名

1247

其ノ人名ヲ報告スヘシ

關東軍司令官 植田大將

下達法、要旨電報後、印刷交付
配布先、次長、次官、23D、關防、野戰司
部内

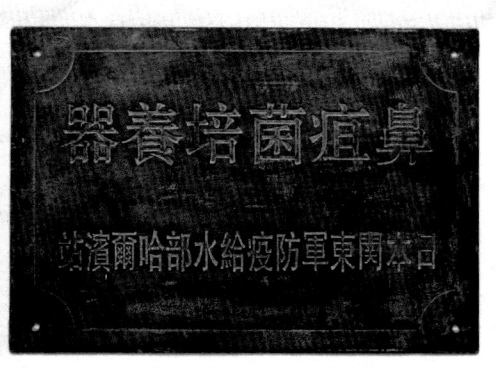

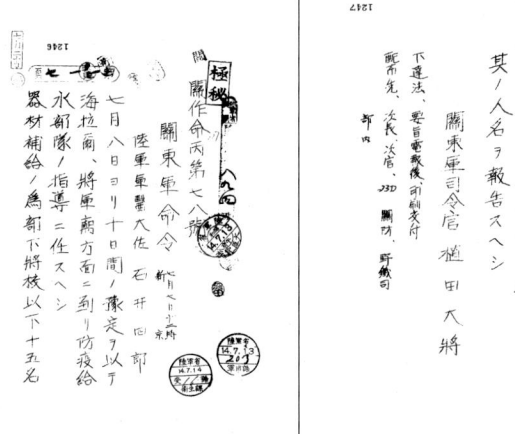

Above left: Fig. 29 Incubator for glanders.

Above right: Fig. 30 'Kanto Army Command Number 78'

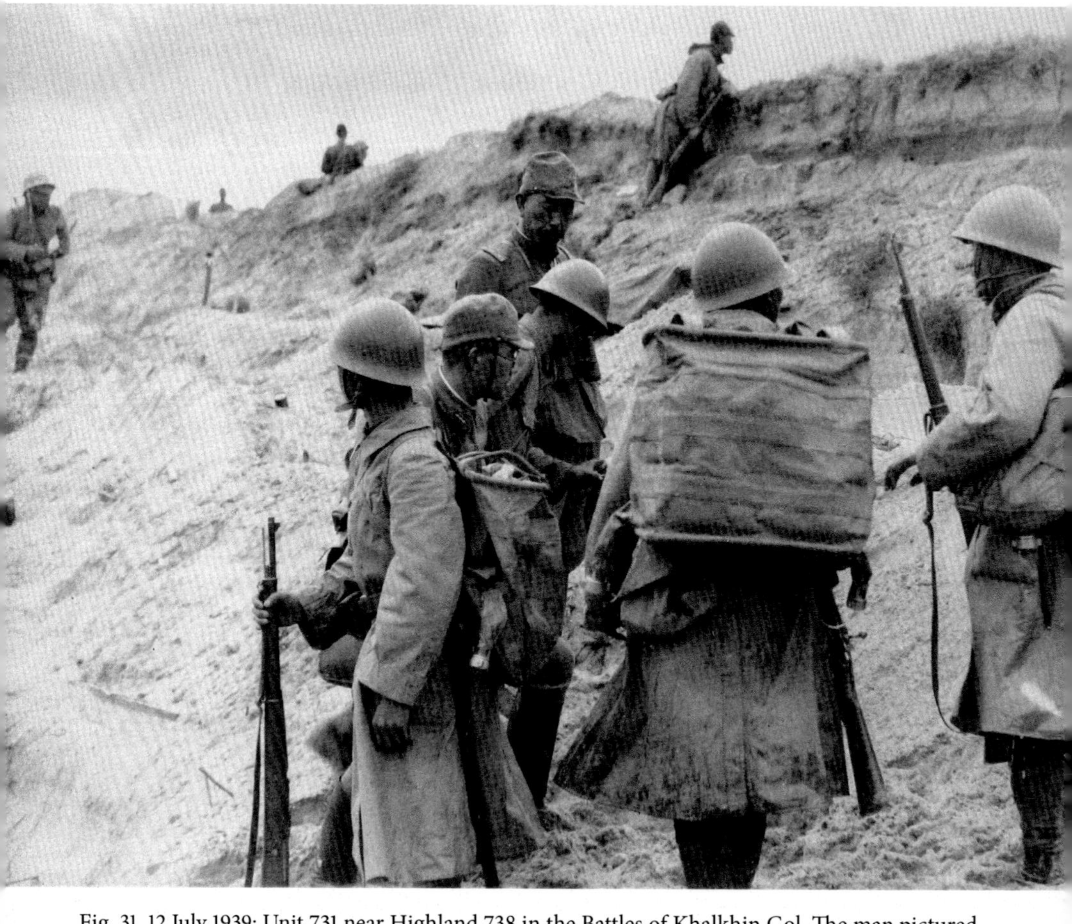

Fig. 31 12 July 1939: Unit 731 near Highland 738 in the Battles of Khalkhin Gol. The man pictured is Shirō Ishii. (*The National Institute for Defense Archive, Japan*)

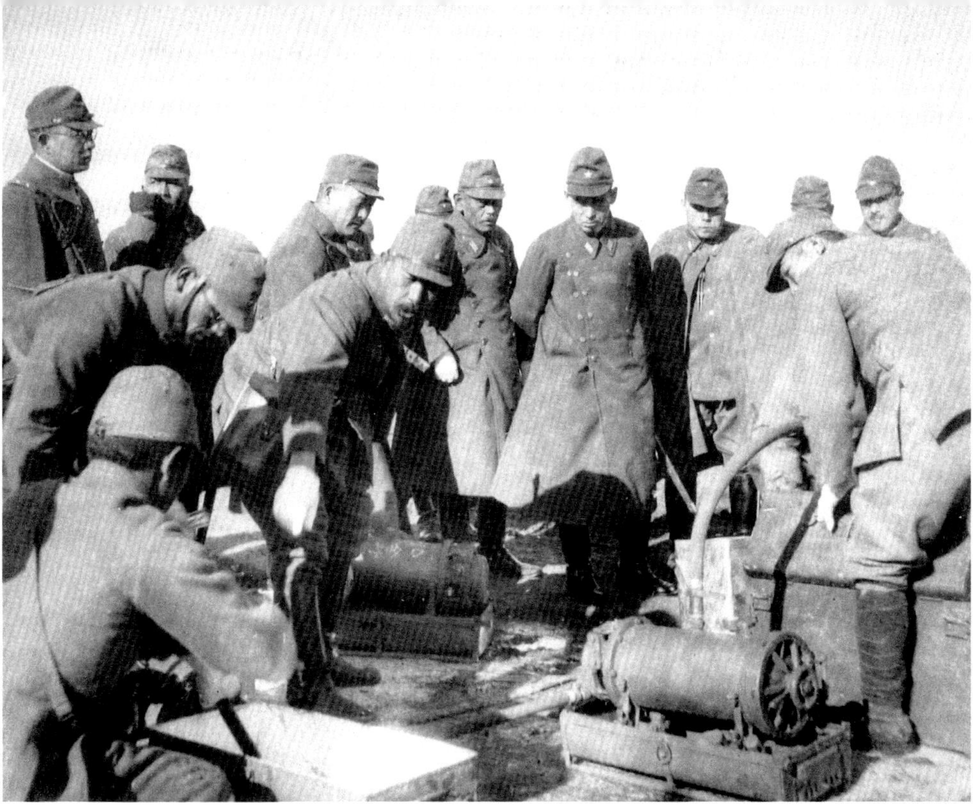

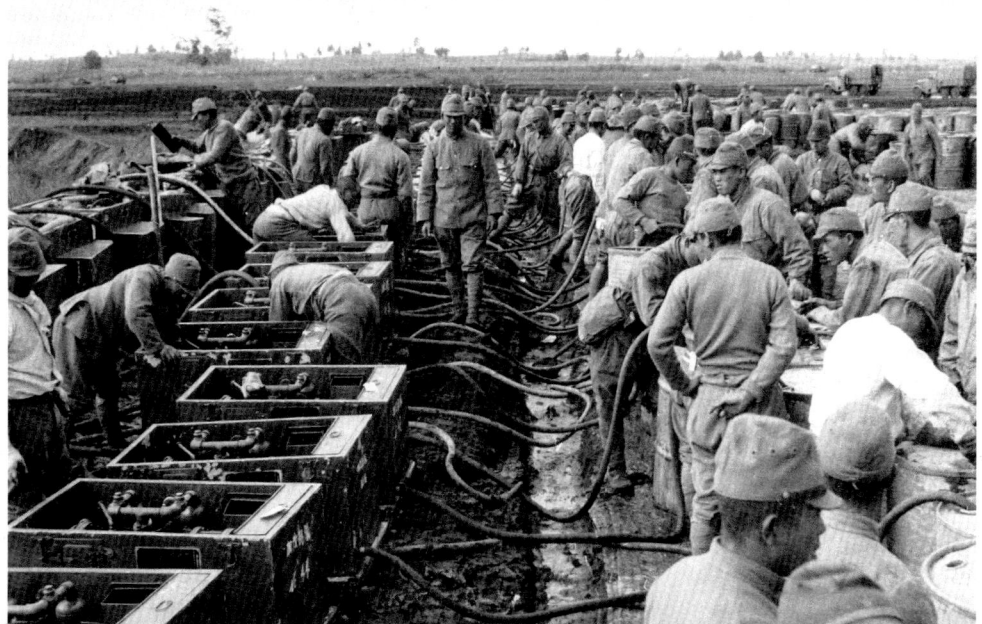

Above: Fig. 32 7 September 1939: Japanese Army Minister Shunroku Hara (the man extending his right hand is Shirō Ishii) inspects Unit 731 in the Battles of Khalkhin Gol. (*The National Institute for Defense Archive, Japan*)

Below: Fig. 33 16 September 1939: Huihe Area in the Battles of Khalkhin Gol. (*The National Institute for Defense Archive, Japan*)

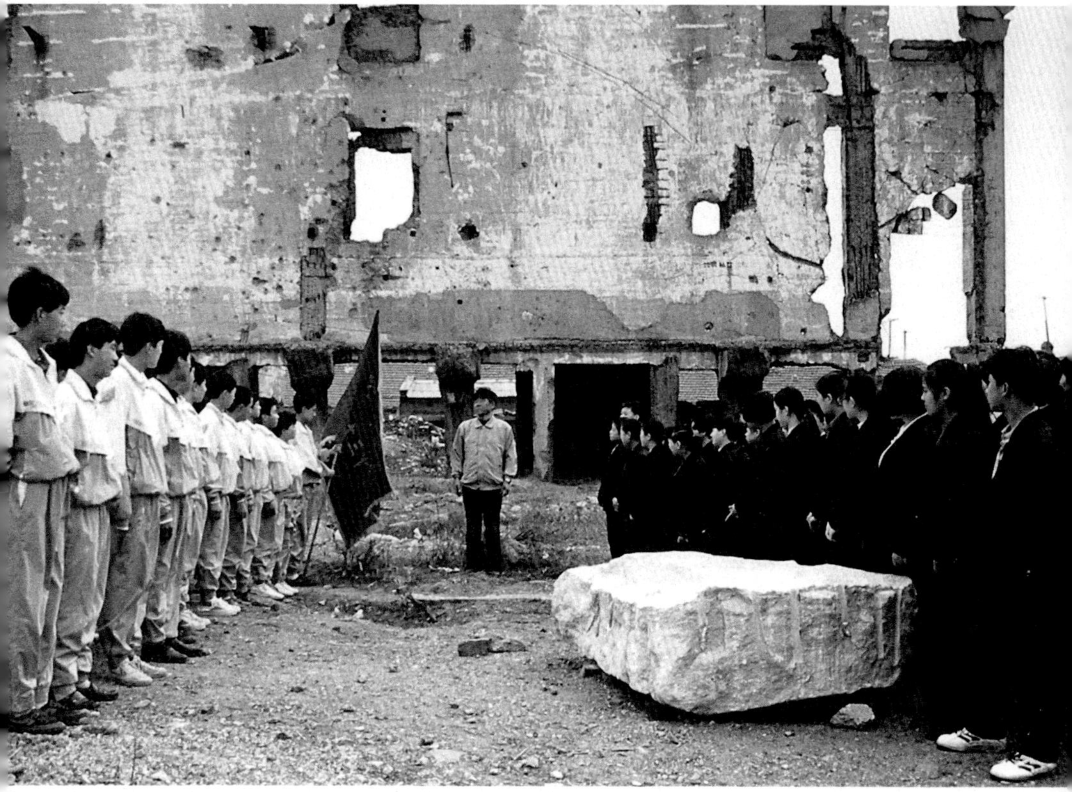

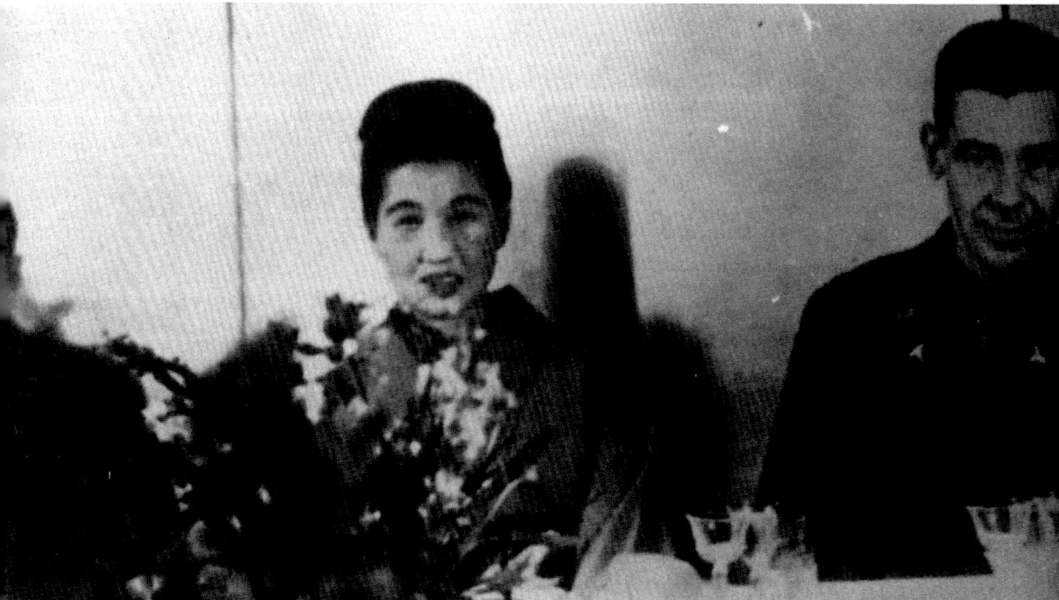

Fig. 34 Fuhe Jing (middle) shares his family story with secondary school students in front of the former boiler room of Unit 731.

Fig. 35 Thompson (left) conducting interrogation in Shirō Ishii's home. The woman is Ishii's wife, Kiyoko Ishii.

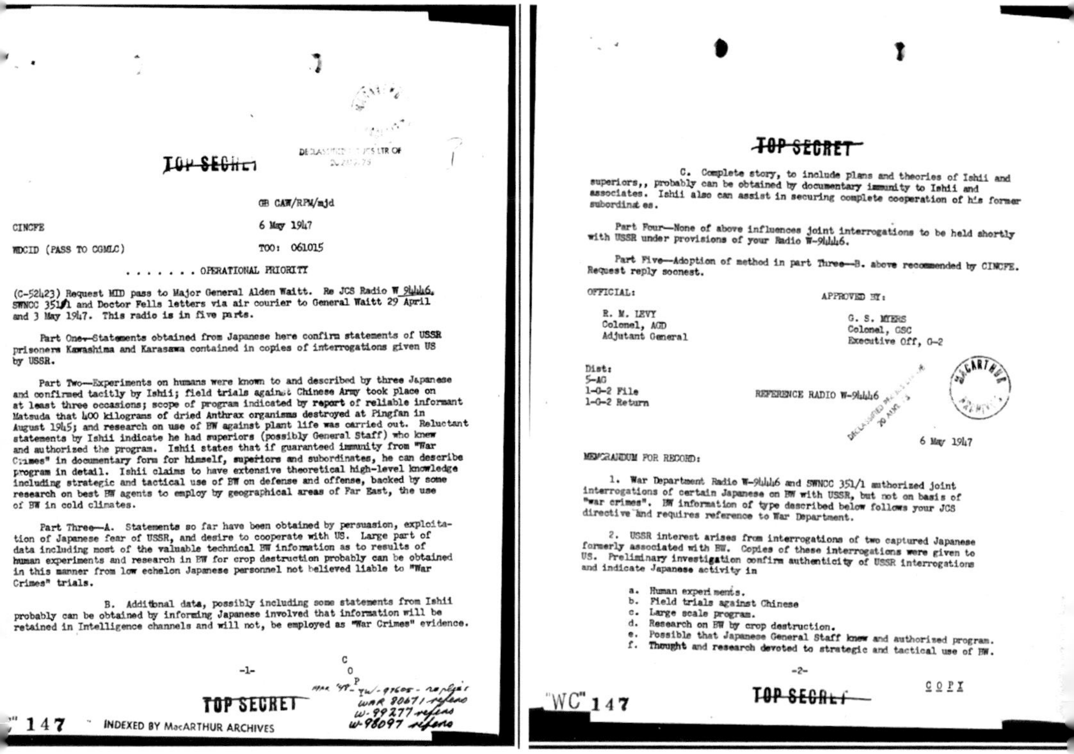

GB CAW/RPM/mjd

CINCFE   6 May 1947

WDCID (PASS TO CGMLC)   TOO: 061015

. . . . OPERATIONAL PRIORITY

(C-52423) Request MID pass to Major General Alden Waitt. Re JCS Radio W-94446. SWNCC 351/1 and Doctor Fells letters via air courier to General Waitt 29 April and 3 May 1947. This radio is in five parts.

Part One—Statements obtained from Japanese here confirm statements of USSR prisoners Kawashima and Karasawa contained in copies of interrogations given US by USSR.

Part Two—Experiments on humans were known to and described by three Japanese and confirmed tacitly by Ishii; field trials against Chinese Army took place on at least three occasions; scope of program indicated by report of reliable informant Matsuda that 400 kilograms of dried Anthrax organisms destroyed at Pingfan in August 1945; and research on use of BW against plant life was carried out. Reluctant statements by Ishii indicate he had superiors (possibly General Staff) who knew and authorized the program. Ishii states that if guaranteed immunity from "War Crimes" in documentary form for himself, superiors and subordinates, he can describe program in detail. Ishii claims to have extensive theoretical high-level knowledge including strategic and tactical use of BW on defense and offense, backed by some research on best BW agents to employ by geographical areas of Far East, the use of BW in cold climates.

Part Three—A. Statements so far have been obtained by persuasion, exploitation of Japanese fear of USSR, and desire to cooperate with US. Large part of data including most of the valuable technical BW information as to results of human experiments and research in BW for crop destruction probably can be obtained in this manner from low echelon Japanese personnel not believed liable to "War Crimes" trials.

B. Additional data, possibly including some statements from Ishii probably can be obtained by informing Japanese involved that information will be retained in Intelligence channels and will not, be employed as "War Crimes" evidence.

-1-

"147"   INDEXED BY MacARTHUR ARCHIVES

C. Complete story, to include plans and theories of Ishii and superiors, probably can be obtained by documentary immunity to Ishii and associates. Ishii also can assist in securing complete cooperation of his former subordinates.

Part Four—None of above influences joint interrogations to be held shortly with USSR under provisions of your Radio W-94446.

Part Five—Adoption of method in part Three—B. above recommended by CINCFE. Request reply soonest.

OFFICIAL: APPROVED BY:

R. M. LEVY   G. S. MYERS
Colonel, AGD   Colonel, GSC
Adjutant General   Executive Off, G-2

Dist:
5-AG
1-G-2 File   REFERENCE RADIO W-94446
1-G-2 Return

6 May 1947

MEMORANDUM FOR RECORD:

1. War Department Radio W-94446 and SWNCC 351/1 authorized joint interrogations of certain Japanese on BW with USSR, but not on basis of "war crimes". BW information of type described below follows your JCS directive and requires reference to War Department.

2. USSR interest arises from interrogations of two captured Japanese formerly associated with BW. Copies of these interrogations were given to US. Preliminary investigation confirm authenticity of USSR interrogations and indicate Japanese activity in

a. Human experiments.
b. Field trials against Chinese
c. Large scale program.
d. Research on BW by crop destruction.
e. Possible that Japanese General Staff knew and authorized program.
f. Thought and research devoted to strategic and tactical use of BW.

-2-

"WC"147   C O P Y

Above: Fig. 36 Documents of exchange between Japan and the US. (*National Archives and Records Administration Archives II*)

Below: Fig. 37 Aerial image of the former Unit 731, photo shot in August 1940.

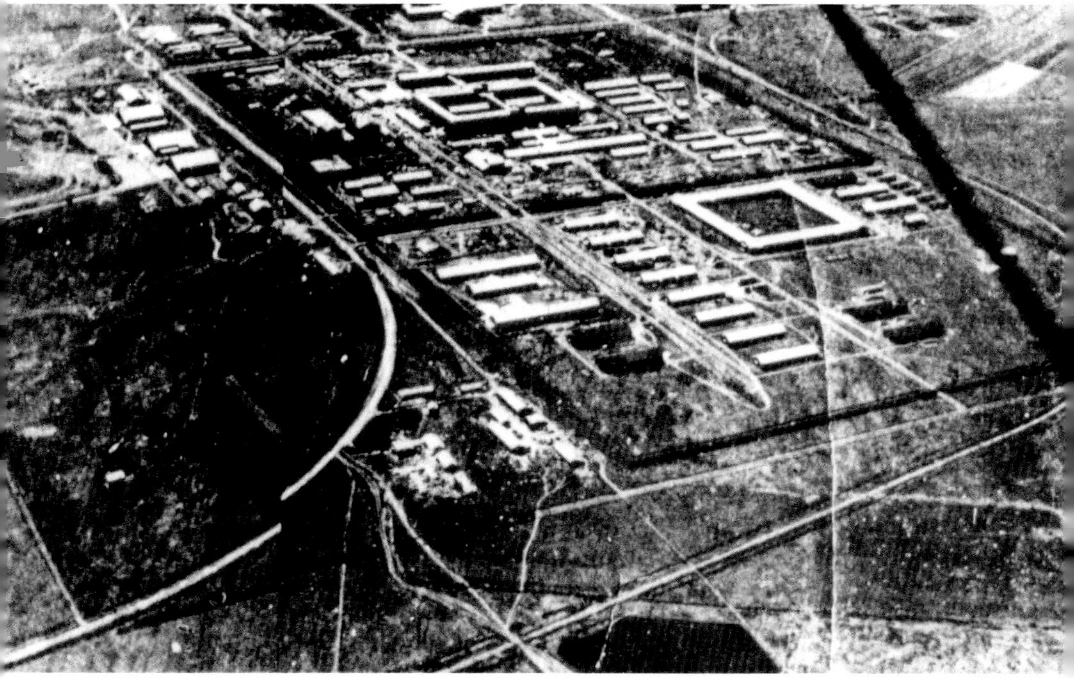

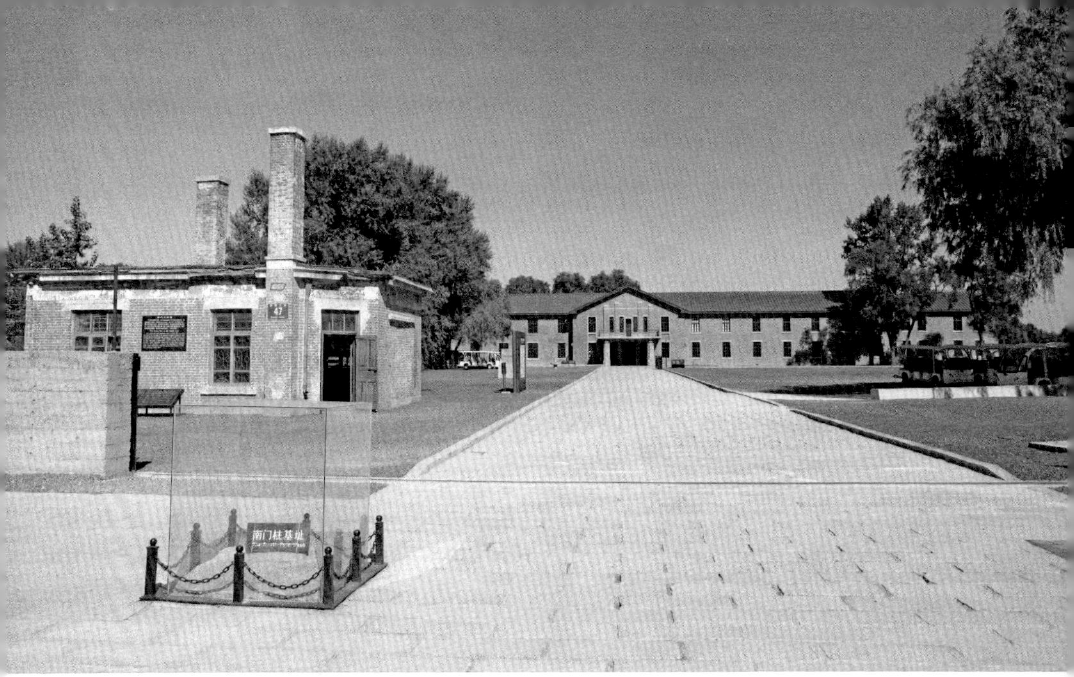

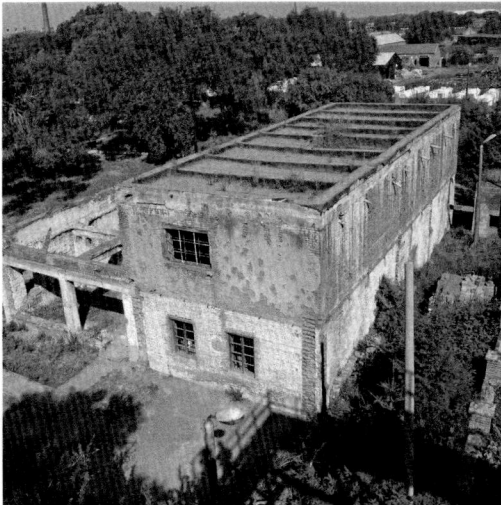

Fig 38 Sites of the main building and south guard gate. (*2015, property of the Museum of War Crime Evidence by Japanese Army Unit 731*)

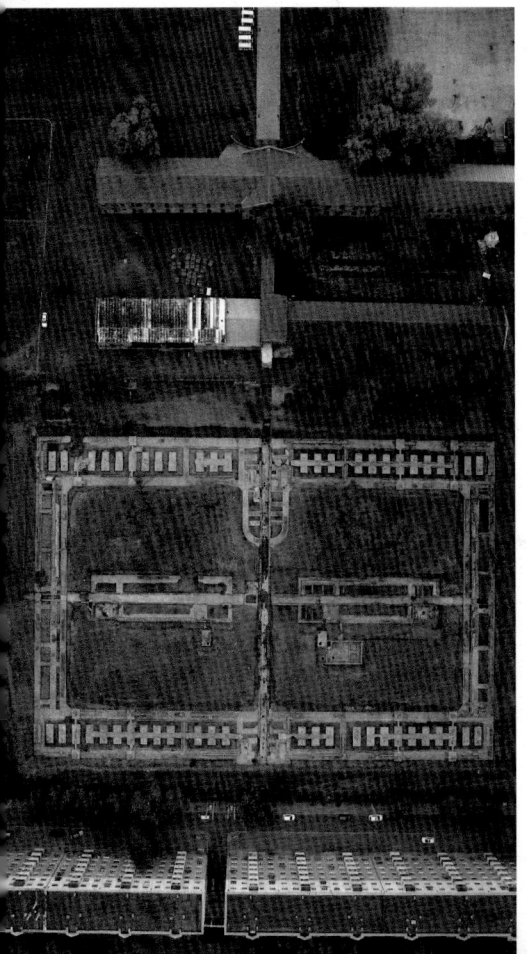

Above: Fig. 39 Site of the frostbite laboratory in 2012. (*Yang Yanjun*)

Left: Fig. 40 Aerial image of the former Sifanglou in Unit 731. (*2015, property of the Museum of War Crime Evidence by Japanese Army Unit 731*)

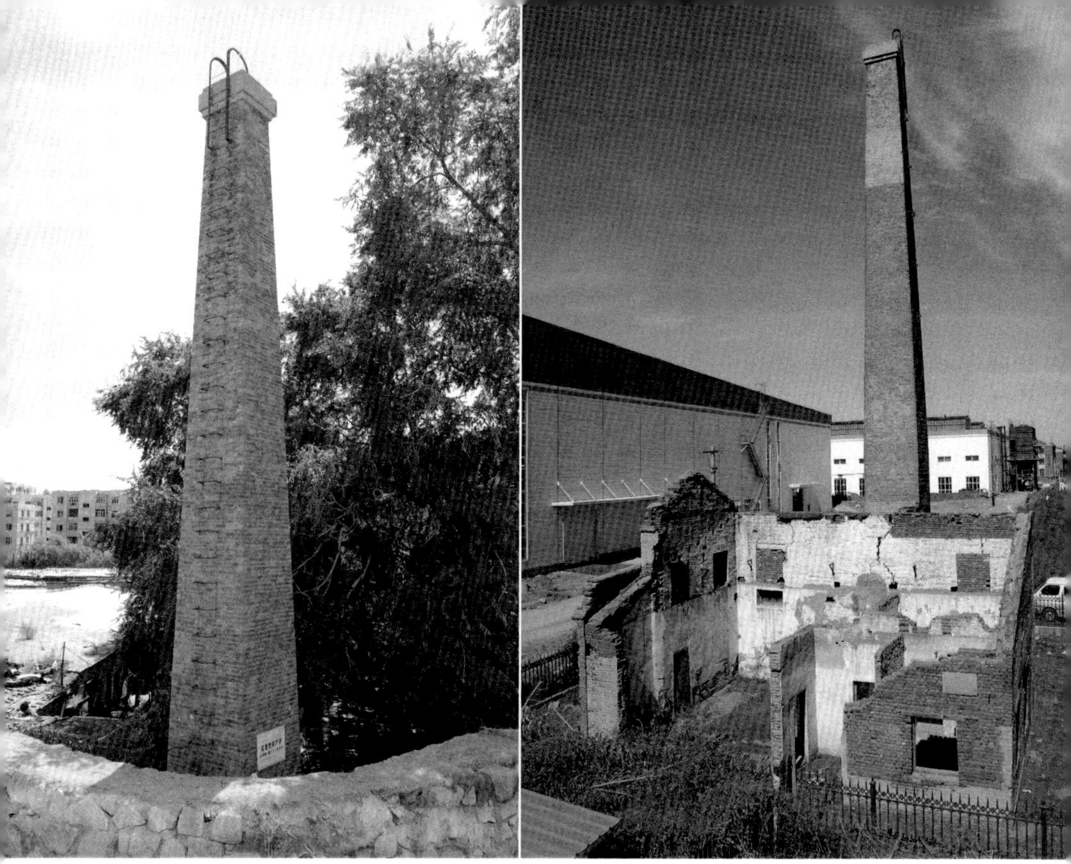

Above: Fig. 41 Former sites of Beiwadi (left) and Beigang (right) crematories. (*2012, photo by Cheng Zhang, Yan-jun Yang*)

Below: Fig. 42 The former site of ground squirrel breeding room. (*2012, photo taken by Wenjing Gong*)

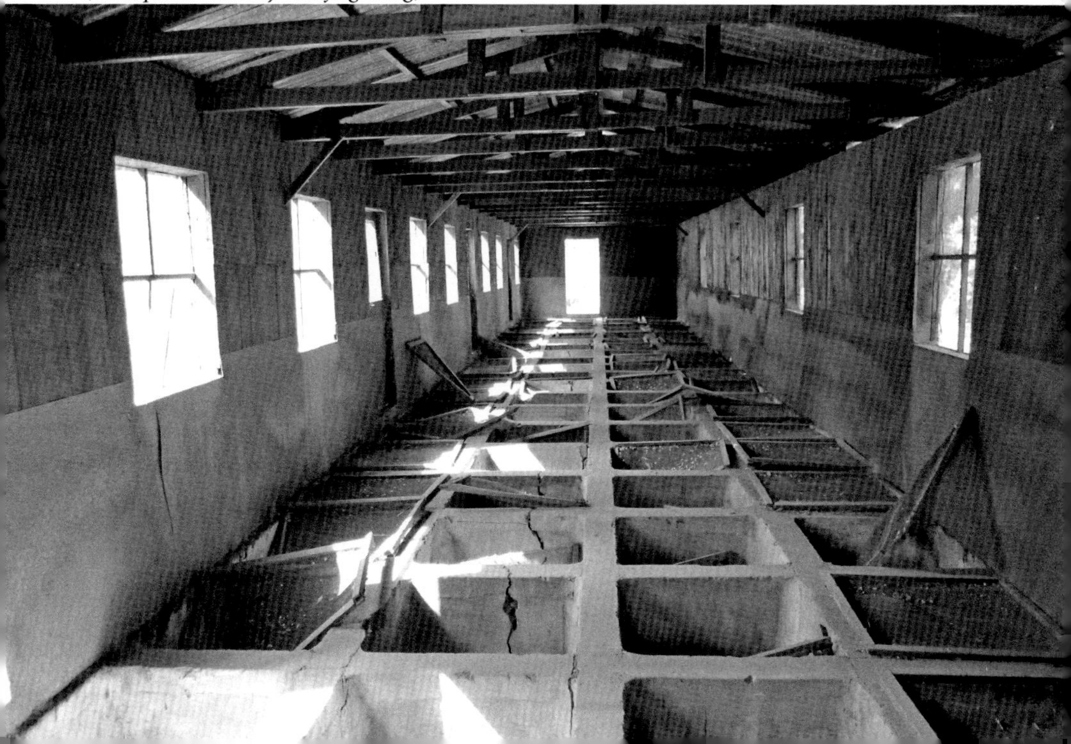

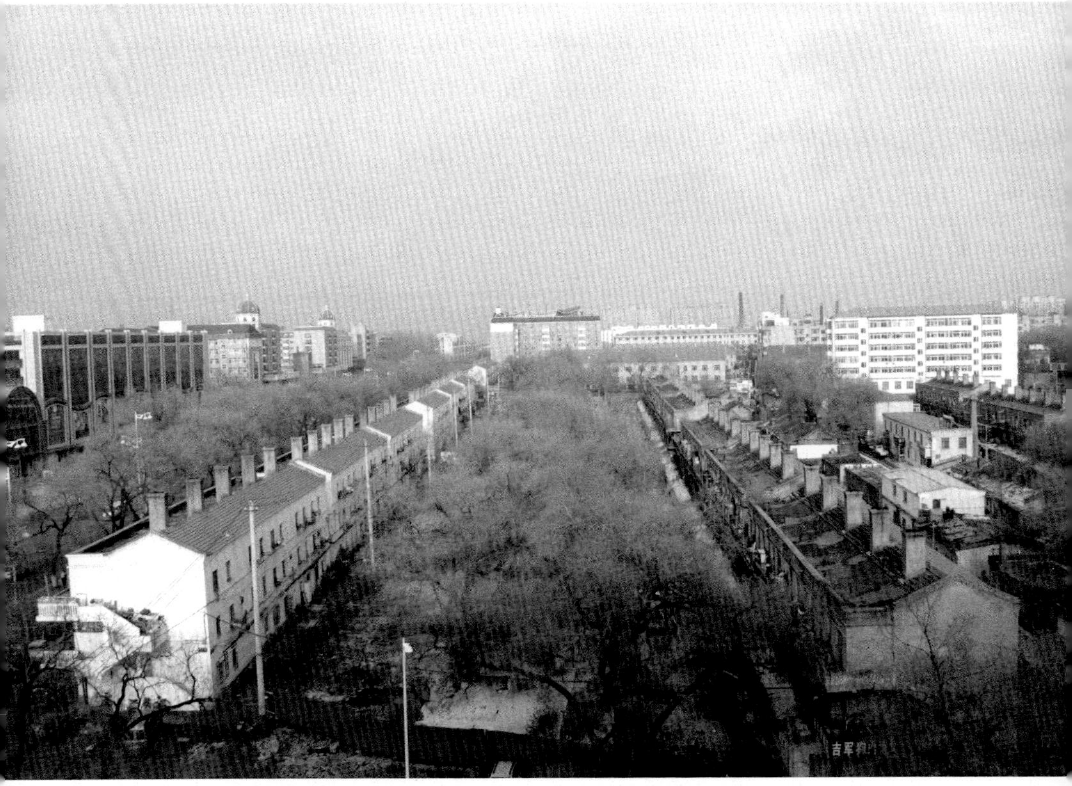

Fig. 43 Former dormitories of Unit 731. (*2012, photo by Han Huiguang*)

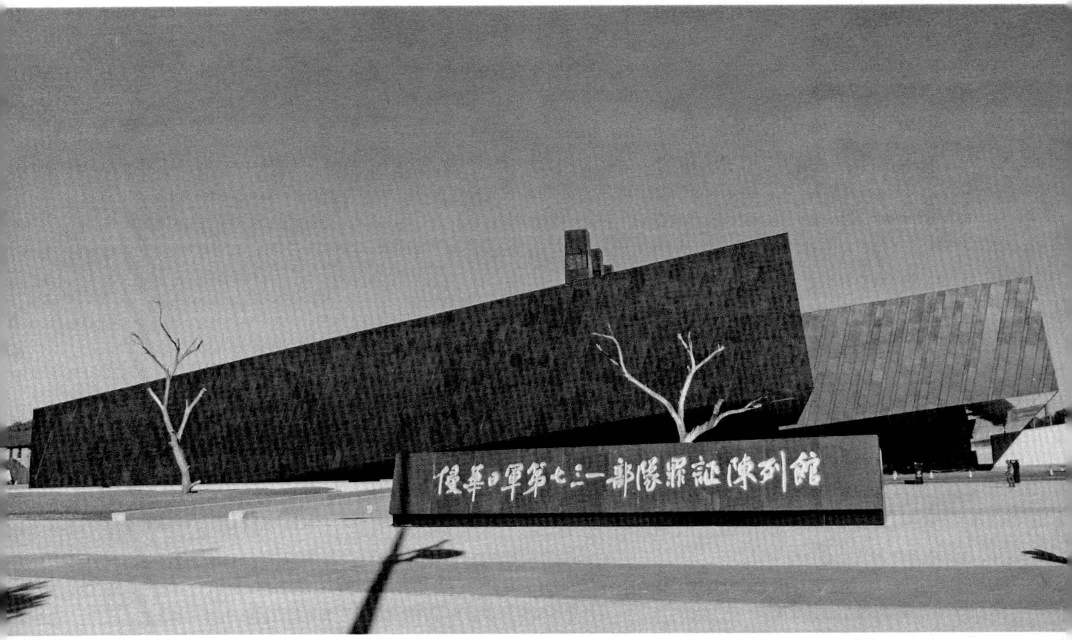

侵华日军第七三一部队罪证陈列馆

Fig. 44 New Building of the Museum of War Crime Evidence by Japanese Army Unit 731. (*2015, property of the Museum of War Crime Evidence by Japanese Army Unit 731*)

A: When those experiments came up, a number of men from each group were picked out to do the work. They were only together temporarily and were disbanded when the experiment was completed.

Q: Were all the people in such groups informed of the nature of the work?

A: They were not informed of what they were doing. They protested that they could not carry on with their own experiments and that their regular work was being interfered with.

Q: Would not more progress have been made if those working on the experiment had been told what it was all about?

A: If they had known what they were working on they would have shrunk up from fright and asked for more pay. They were not well-trained men

Q: A soldier is a soldier and could you not have ordered them to do the work?

A: They were not soldiers. They were reservists. Those in the branch units were soldiers, but not those in the main unit. I could not order them.

Q: How much research cooperation was given by the Navy on BW?

A: There was no cooperation whatsoever.[13] [See Fig. 35.]

At the time of this interrogation, the Tokyo Trials had started. Whether to work with the US Army or not, and in what ways, were key factors that would impact the destiny of Shirō Ishii and his team members in Unit 731. Ishii was receiving a high volume of interrogation in the Trials. The investigation by the US Army affected Shirō Ishii, but he did not deny or fully admit his responsibility in Unit 731.

In order to conceal his crimes and avoid trial and sentencing, Ishii deflected the US Army interrogators. Under investigation, he covered up the facts of Japanese biological warfare, biological weapons, and human experimentation and only admitted involvement in bacterial and preventive medical research.

At the same time, he led Thompson into the sensitive topic of Soviet biological warfare preparation, with which he tried to complicate the issue of biological warfare. Thompson's report above shows the US Army failed to gain what was expected from Shirō Ishii.

Thompson's Assessment of Ishii

Shirō Ishii attempted to deflect Thompson's first investigation, however, his plan to escape the Tokyo Trials was known to Thompson. In subsequent reports, Thompson said:

The information regarding Japanese BW activities obtained from presumably independent sources was consistent to the point where it seems that the informants had been instructed as to the amount and nature of information that was to be divulged under interrogation.

All information was presumably furnished from memory since all records are said to have been destroyed in accordance with directives of the Japanese Amy. Yet, some of the information, especially sketches of the bombs, was in such detail as to question the contention that all documentary evidence had been destroyed. It was evident throughout the interrogations that it was the desire of the Japanese to minimise the extent of their activities in BW, especially the effort devoted to offensive research and development.[14]

In general, the previous three points by Thompson are accurate. He discovered that immediately prior to the beginning of war crimes investigation, Ishii and other members secretly agreed not to reveal the truth.

During the US investigation into Japanese biological warfare, Ishii's assistant, Ryoichi Naito, who had been in charge of the disease prevention centre, took action to contact the US Army. During negotiations with the Army, Naito revealed details heard from the US Army to other Unit 731 members. Thompson doubted the validity of the destruction of all information by the Japanese Army, and he believed Ishii hid facts about the creation of biological weapons. Based on the preceding narrative, Thompson was dissatisfied with what he heard, and he then aimed to interrogate Masaji Kitano, who had just escaped to Japan from China. Ishii and Kitano were core members of Unit 731, and Thompson's intent was to gain as much evidence as he could from major participants.

The Unit 731 facilities had vanished, but once its members escaped to Japan, they set up operation headquarters in Noma Shrine (野間神社) in Kanazawa. Most of the research information bought from Unit 731 in Harbin was kept in this Noma Shrine. The order for secrecy given by Shirō Ishii remained in effect among former members, and as commander, he used his position to fabricate the same narrative for other members. At the same time, he requested members investigate the information sought by the US Army. While he did not fully understand the aim of the US investigation, he feared he would be sent to the Tokyo Trials if the US Army did not believe his testimony.

Completion of Thompson's Report

From 5 February to 11 March 1946, Thompson conducted interrogation of Shirō Ishii and other members and completed his 'Report about Japanese Biological Weapons' on 31 May 1947.[15] The forty-eight-page report includes Shirō's biography, educational background, and record of overseas trips for biological warfare research, as well as the organisation, management, and duties of Unit 731.

Through 'The Thompson Report', Shirō Ishii provided useful material that allowed the US to learn about human resource management, organisation, research areas, and progress, as well as bacteriological warfare and human experimentation. He responded more fully to Thompson's investigation than he did to Sanders. At the beginning, he refused to discuss bacteriological warfare and human experimentation, but later he welcomed Thompson's questions regarding these sensitive issues. The reason for his change of attitude remains unknown. In my opinion, he could have known that 'the investigation would not be used as evidence in war trials'.[16]

The following are Shirō Ishii's points as reported by Thompson:

Failure to fully utilise Japanese scientific capability by restriction of BW research and development to the military with lack of cooperation between the military services precluded progress toward development of BW into a practical weapon. Had a practical BW weapon been achieved, it is unlikely that Japan would have resorted to its use because of fear retaliation by means of chemical warfare. Insofar as could be learned, Japan had no information of American activity in BW.[17]

According to current information, research on biological weapons by Unit 731 was supported by the Japanese Military Department, the Japanese Army, Kanto Army, and some other institutions, such as Tokyo Army Surgeon Hospital School, Kanto Army Unit 100, and Unit 516. At the same time, Tokyo Imperial University, Kyoto Imperial University, and some other Japanese medical schools provided support and assistance to Unit 731, which allowed the Unit to build powerful connections with top research institutions from military and medical fields. In 'The Thompson Report', Thompson revealed his lack of understanding the truth of Japanese research on biological weapons, and at the same time admitted that the US was involved in the same kind of research.

Investigation by Norbert Fell

On 4 April 1947, Cdr Alden Waitt of the US Biological Warfare Unit sent Norbert Fell to Tokyo to investigate Japanese biological warfare. Fell was an expert in microbiology and epidemiology, a graduate of the University of Chicago, and head of the plant laboratory at the Detrick military base.

Interrogation by United States Department of Defense

Fell arrived in Tokyo on 13 April 1947 and interrogated members of Unit 731 previously investigated by Sanders and Thompson. Fell received a telegram from United State Department of Defense on 15 May 1947 that held questions from Dr Norman to Fell:

Part 1:   What were the main crops considered by the Japanese group concerned with crop destruction?

Part 2:   What plant diseases, organisms, or insects were studied?

Part 3:   Was the intent to attack by sabotage or by direct application of the agent to the crop by airplane?

Part 4:   Where was the laboratory work carried out? What sort of facilities did the laboratories have?

Part 5:   Who were the chief technical people involved, and what positions had they held previously?

Part 6:   Were field trials carried out? On a small plot basis or on a large scale? Were any of these in isolated areas or on islands?

Part 7:   How was it proposed to distribute the agents for crops? By dropping test tube cultures, or use of bombs or sprays from airplanes? If either of the latter, what kind of equipment was developed?

Part 8:   Was attention given to defensive measures, such as spraying of crops that had previously been treated?

Part 9:   Were any experiments carried out on effects on crops of chemicals such as oil, war gases, or poisons or weed killers?

Part 10: Were experiments carried out on burning of crops or vegetation by incendiaries and/or spraying or treating?

Part 11: Were there any gardens or field plots at or near the BW installation? How big were they? Were they isolated from other farms? What crops were growing?

Part 12: Did you see men working in the plots, spraying or dusting the plants? Did any of the crops die or change color? Did airplanes fly over them at low altitude?

Part 13: Do you know if grain or vegetables from these plots were fed to animals or men.

Part 14: Were there any agronomists, plant pathologists, botanists, crop breeders. Or entomologists on the technical staff of the BW installation? What sort of work were they doing?

Part 15: Were chemical weed killers in use in Japan before the war? If so, what substances were used? Were they available during the war?

Part 16: What crop diseases do you know of or can recognise? Do any of these cause series loses in the vicinity of the BW installation?[18]

Fell interrogated Shirō Ishii, Tomohisa Masuda, Junichi Kaneko, Ryoichi Naito, Wakamatsu Arijirou, and a few others and included the transcript in 'The Latest Information on Japanese Biological Warfare Activity', also known as 'The Fell Report', on 20 June 1947.[19] This report is kept in the National Archives in Maryland, US.

Chief Content of 'The Fell Report'
According to the report, there was a special notice on 'The Fell Report':

Anyone who received this attachment must sign in the blank at left. Anyone who knows about the content of this attachment has to sign the blank on the right. Only the last person who receives this attachment has the right to distribute this attachment when highly necessary. The person needs to keep or return the report and this attachment according to the regulation. This attachment must remain with the report until this report is returned to the top-secret document keeper. According to Information Security Department document number 380–5 passage 26, this attachment needs to be transferred by specially appointed respondent. When the attachment is unused, it should be kept in a safety box with three locks or similar security box. There should be a receipt during the postage process [this attachment is equivalent to a receipt]. When the document is not in the post, it should be managed by top secret document keepers or top secret document assistants. The decryption of documents is decided by The United States Department of Defense. The class of decryption is adjusted in every three years. Decryption will be released after 12 years. This document is currently decrypted.[20]

Human Experimentation: 'The Fell Report' recorded the result of human experimentation of anthrax, plague, typhoid fever, dysentery, cholera, and glanders conducted by Unit 731. This comprises approximately 70 per cent of the report.

Plant Biological Warfare: 'The Fell Report' details information about plant biological warfare of Unit 731, as well as the relationship between plant biological warfare and agronomists, biologists and entomologists. Information related to prevention and effects on humans and animals is also included in the report.

Article by Shirō Ishii: According to 'The Fell Report', Ishii wrote an article about Japanese biological warfare's entire scope, summarising his twenty years of experiments on biological warfare, his ideas on the use of biological weapons and war strategy, and how the weapons function under different environmental conditions, especially in extremely cold weather. Unfortunately, this report did not include the complete article, which certainly exists somewhere in the US.

Barrage Balloons: 'The Fell Report' recorded information about barrage balloons invented by the Japanese for attacking the US from 1942 to 1945. These barrage balloons were one weapon that bought threat and fear to the US. Unit 731 was involved in the research of barrage balloons and attempted to use barrage balloons to spread biological threats and bacteria.

Fell stated in his report that most of the research conducted by the US Army at the Detrick base had also been researched by the Japanese.

Investigation by Hill and Victor

In October 1947, Dr Edwin V. Hill and Dr Joseph Victor were sent from the Detrick base to Japan to investigate Japanese biological warfare. Hill was director of the experiment department at Detrick, and Victor was a pathologist. From 29 October to 25 November 1947, Hill and Victor interrogated Shirō Ishii, Masaji Kitano, Tomohisa Masuda, and nineteen others. They released 'Summary Report on B.W. Investigations', also known as 'Hill's Report', based on their interrogation and submitted it to the US Department of Defense in December 1947.

The aim of 'Hill's Report' was to fill in gaps left in earlier investigations by Sanders, Thompson, and Fell and to provide additional information about Unit 731. At the conclusion, Hill wrote:

Evidence gathered in this investigation has greatly supplemented and amplified previous aspects of this field. It represents data which have been obtained by

Japanese scientists at the expenditure of many millions of dollars and years of work. Information has accrued with respect to human susceptibility to these diseases as indicated by specific infectious doses of bacteria. Such information could not be obtained in our own laboratories because of scruples attached to human experimentation. These data were occurred with a total outlay of ¥ 250,000 to date, a more pittance by comparison with the actual cost of the studies.[21]

Secret Deal between the US and Japan

Telegrams between Washington and Tokyo

On 7 February 1947, the inspector of Soviet Union requested permission from the International Military Tribunal for the Far East to interrogate Shirō Ishii, Hitoshi Kikuchi, and Masumi Ota. The Soviet attitude toward members of Unit 731 differed from that of the US.

Gen. Douglas MacArthur sent the following telegram to the Washington Joint Staff:

> Request based on information alleged to have been obtained from unidentified prisoners of war who stated that experiments authorised and conducted by above three Japanese resulted in deaths of 2000 Chinese and Manchurians. Russians present request on their assumption that supplementary war crimes trials will be authorised by United States, but also admit interest in mass production of typhus and cholera bacteria and typhus bearing fleas at PINGFAN said to have been described by prisoners of war to them. Opinion here that Russian not likely to obtain information form Japanese not already known to United States and that United States might get some additional information from Russian line of questioning in monitored interrogations.[22]

On 21 March, the Washington Joint Staff replied by telegram to Gen. Douglas MacArthur: 'Based on the following factors, the Soviet Union is approved to interrogate Shirō Ishii, Army Colonel Masumi Ota and Hitoshi Kikuchi about biological warfare.[23] … Before the interrogation, it is a must to inform the Japanese experts of biological warfare not to mention the US interrogation to the Soviet Union'.[24]

The US agreed to allow the Soviet Union to investigate regarding biological warfare, but in order to keep the information to themselves, the US discussed with Ishii and the other members not to disclose any detail of the US investigation or any important information regarding biological warfare to the Soviet Union.

This act is the same as the US investigation of the members of Unit 731—compromise before providing declarations.

The Secret Deal in the Telegram

On 6 May 1947, the Supreme Commander for the Allied Powers sent an urgent telegram, no. 52423, to the US Department of Defense. It contained five parts:

Statements obtained from Japanese here confirm statements of USSR prisoners Kawashima and Karasawa contained in copies of interrogations given US by USSR.

Experiments on humans were known to and described by three Japanese and confirmed tacitly by Ishii; field trials against Chinese Army took place on at least three occasions; scope of program indicated by report of reliable informant Matsuda that 400 kilograms of dried Anthrax organisms destroyed at Pingfang in August 1945; and research on use of BW against plant life was carried out. Reluctant statements by Ishii indicate he had superiors [possibly General Staff] who knew and authorized the program. Ishii states that if guaranteed immunity from 'War Crimes' in documentary form for himself, superiors and subordinates, he can describe program in detail. Ishii claims to have extensive theoretical high-level knowledge including strategic and tactical use of BW on defense and offense, backed by some research on best BW agents to employ by geographical areas of Far East, the use of BW in cold climates.

(A) Statements so far have been obtained by persuasion, exploitation of Japanese fear of USSR, and desire to cooperate with US. Large part of data including most of the valuable technical BW information as to results of human experiments and research in BW for crop destruction probably can be obtained in this manner from low echelon Japanese personnel not believed liable to 'War Crimes' Trials.

(B) Additional data, possibly including some statements from Ishii probably can be obtained by informing Japanese involved that information will be retained in Intelligence channels and will not, be employed as 'War Crimes' evidence.

(C) Complete story, to include plans and theories of Ishii and superiors, probably can be obtained by documentary immunity to Ishii and associates. Ishii also can assist in securing complete cooperation of his former subordinates.

None of above influences joint interrogations to be held shortly with USSR under provisions of your Radio W-94446.

Adoption of method in part Three-B. above recommended by CINCFE. Request reply soonest.[25] [See Fig. 36.]

'... could inform the Japanese that, the related information would be kept as important source and would not be used as war crime evidence in the Trial'.

This is US Forces in Japan's suggestion to the US Department of Defense in order to collect information and data on biological warfare and human experimentation, and they also suggested that 'Plans and information from Shirō Ishii and his higher authorities may collected by exempting them from trial in written form'.[26]

It is hard to follow all comments from the Washington headquarters in 1946 and 1947, but simply put, the Supreme Commander of the Allied Powers was able to use all means and methods to investigate Japan, Unit 731, and war-related individuals in order to collect information beneficial to the US.

During the investigation and interrogation of members of Unit 731, the US implied to members of Unit 731 that their disclosures would not be used as evidence in the Tokyo Trial. Investigators were scientists and experts mainly from the Detrick military base, and the content of investigations was mostly related to biological weapons, strategies of biological warfare and results of experiments.

I suspect that from the beginning of these interrogations, the US focused on acquiring technical information regarding biological warfare, and had no concern whether the information would be used as evidence in the Trial.

United States Department of Defense Concerns

The US Department of Defense sent a telegram to the Supreme Commander of the Allied Powers Law Department on 3 June 1947:

> ... all evidence and information provided by Shirō Ishii and members of his division must be provided to the States in a telegram as soon as possible, especially evidence from Shirō Ishii and his members that the US agreed to exempt them from trial in written form. Which countries among our allies accuse Shirō Ishii and his members? Are Shirō Ishii and his members included in the list of war criminals waiting to undergo trial?[27]

The Supreme Commander of the Allied Powers Law Department replied to the United States Department of Defense on 6 June 1947:

1. The reports and files of the Legal Section on Ishii and his co-workers are based on anonymous letters, hearsay affidavits and rumours. The Legal Section interrogations, to date, of the numerous persons concerned with the BW project in China, do not reveal sufficient evidence to support war crime charges. The alleged victims are of unknown identity. Unconfirmed allegations are to the effect that criminals, farmers, women and children were used for BW experimental purposes. The Japanese communist party alleges that: 'Ishii BKA' [Bacterial War Army] conducted experiments on captured Americans in Mukden and that simultaneously, research on similar lines was conducted in Tokyo and Kyoto.
2. None of Ishii's subordinates are charged or held as war crime suspects, nor is there sufficient evidence on file against them. Ishii's possible superiors, who are now on trial before IMTFF, include Umezu, Commander, Kwantung Army, 1939–44, Minami, Commander, Kwantung Army 1934–36, Koiso, Chief of Staff, Kwantung Army 1932–34, Tojo, Chief of Staff, Kwantung Army 1937–38.
3. None of our Allies to date have filed war crimes charges against Ishii or any of his associates.

4. Neither Ishii nor his associates are included among major Japanese war criminals awaiting trial.[28]

On 22 June 1947, the US Department of Defense requested further information from the Supreme Commander for the Allied Powers:

> … evidence now in its possession warrants opinion that Japanese BW group headed by Ishii did violate rules of land warfare. We are satisfied evidence now in possession Legal Sect SCAP does not warrant such charge against and trial of Ishii and his group. Must have info re all possible proof re Ishii BW group participation in activities that could be considered War Crimes under rules of land warfare before reaching decision reurad C 52423 dtd 6 May 47.[29]

Even though the US understood Ishii's actions were war crimes, the evidence further confirms he was not to be accused and undergo trial or be on the list of war criminals. In order to prevent Ishii's evidence being disclosed in public, the US deliberately ignored the culpability of Unit 731 and Japanese troops. Regarding this, although the US agreed with the suggestions in the telegram of 6 May, there were still concerns.

On 27 June 1947, the Supreme Commander for the Allied Powers Law Department sent an urgent telegram to the Department of Defense providing details from a report that investigated Unit 731 for war crimes, and concluded that 'Japanese BW group headed by ISHII did violate rules of land warfare, but this expression of opinion is not a recommendation that group be charged and tried for such'.[30]

Instruction from the Joint Chiefs of Staff

The Joint Chiefs of Staff sent an order to Douglas MacArthur on 13 March 1948 in reply to telegram no. 52423 of 6 May 1947. The swift reply that MacArthur had requested in his telegram took ten months. The content of the telegram is as follows:

> Reports by technical experts who have returned from your theatre indicate that to date necessary information and scientific data have been obtained to your satisfaction. Suggest your recommendation Part 3 B and 5 be resubmitted for further consideration if and when you consider necessary.[31]

The telegram proved that the US had already obtained the desired information and scientific data on biological warfare, the goal of the four-year investigation. This was an order given to MacArthur, and could be seen as a final agreement on 'plans and information from Shirō Ishii and his higher authorities may be collected by exempting them from trial in written form'.

Ishii requested exemption from trial, and the US believed this would have a huge impact on US foreign affairs and government. So the headquarters sent a tactful reply to MacArthur. After the US gained information from Ishii and his members, they were free from trial. This telegram is the last confirmation document between Shirō Ishii and the US.

Conclusion

The US and Unit 731 secretly sealed a deal that ignored and covered-up war crimes of unethical human experimentation and biological warfare. As Sheldon H. Harris wrote in *Factories of Death*: 'State, in effect, would go along with the Ishii arrangement, so long as nothing potentially embarrassing to the United States [i.e., the revelation that immunity was being accorded war criminals] was documented'.[32] The US cover-up allowed Shirō Ishii and members of his division to escape the Tokyo Trial, which directly affected the fairness and authority of the Trials. This is grossly unfair to the Chinese, American, Russian, and Korean families whose family members suffered in human experimentation.

Regarding this cover-up, Sanders, involved in the interrogations conducted in Japan, stated:

> The deal was a mistake. But when I made such a suggestion, I did not know that they used live human beings as objects in experiments. When I knew they were making anthrax bombs, there was still time to accuse the Japanese in the Tokyo Trials.[33]

While the US forces planned to keep information on biological warfare to themselves, the Soviet Union also actively attempted to collect it. In 1946, it secretly interrogated former Unit 731 members Kawashima Kiyoshi (川島清) and Tomio Kawakawa (柄澤十三夫).

The issue of Japanese biological warfare became a tug-of-war with the Supreme Commander for the Allied Powers, and the US finally took the lead in the Tokyo Trials in order to continue to conceal the matter of Japanese biological warfare and human experimentation, ignoring the rights of people in China and the Soviet Union.

Persistent Soviet requests to interrogate Japanese war criminals on this topic failed to get a reply from the US, so such interrogation did not take place. The Soviet Union lacked the power to dictate this compared to the US, and this issue did not affect the result of the Tokyo Trials, whose consequences continue today.

The Soviet Union sent twelve Japanese war criminals in biological warfare to Khabarovsk Krai, a far eastern district of Russia.

The content of the trial was published in *Materials on the Trial of Former Servicemen of the Japanese Army Charged with Manufacturing and Employing Bacteriological Weapons*. This publication is translated into Chinese, English, German, Japanese, Korean, and other languages. Reviewing the Soviet Union's trial of Japanese war criminals helps understand the hidden information regarding the covert deals between the US and Japan.

Protection of Sites and Museum

In 1945, just days before the official end of the war, members of Unit 731 destroyed most of the buildings and facilities on the site. Remaining structures were later destroyed by urban development, social changes and natural disasters, business growth and individuals, and other complicated processes. Seventy years later, more than eighty buildings remained, twenty-three of which were designated Major Historical and Cultural Sites Protected at the National Level.

Protection Process

Proper protection of remaining sites of Unit 731 by both central and local governments began in 1950, following the establishment of the People's Republic of China. In the spring of 1956, Zhikun Wang (王之堃) of Harbin produced a film of nine minutes and ten seconds; this was the first documentary showing the ruins remaining after the mass destruction. The surviving sites of Unit 731 were largely destroyed between 1957 and 1981 (see Fig. 37).

In the 1980s, many government-approved Japanese history textbooks omitted the Japanese invasion of China and attempted to whitewash the war crimes committed by the servicemen of the former Japanese imperial forces. This prompted the Chinese to consider the importance of preserving the remains of Unit 731.

In August 1982, an investigative team created by the Harbin government started research on preservation of Unit 731 sites and interviewed war victims. On 17 September, Japanese writer Seiichi Morimura visited the sites and met with Yan Xia (夏衍), the former chair of the Ministry of Culture of the People's Republic of China in Beijing. During the meeting, Morimura made suggestions regarding protection of the ruins, which were taken seriously by the Chinese government.

On 25 December 1982, the Harbin government officially issued an administrative order 'About Protection of the Sites of War Crimes by the Former Japanese Kanto Army', followed by the establishment of the Administration of Cultural Relics of

Pingfang, charged with the clean-up, research, excavation, and organisation of the ruins. This is the first time a Chinese local government mandated protection of relics as a civic duty.

On 7 March 1983, Heilongjiang Province government decreed the former sites of Unit 731 a Major Historical and Cultural Site Protected at the Provincial Level. On 15 August 1985, the museum was opened to the public. From 1991 to 1993, twenty-two areas of ruins were designated as protected areas. On 15 August 1995, a new museum, located 300 metres east of the main building, opened to the public. From 1999 to 2011, 143 residences and twelve public housing units were removed from the site, and eleven areas of ruins (10,400 square metres) were opened.

In 2006, the museum became a Major Historical and Cultural Site Protected at the National Level. In 2011, the city of Harbin announced the Harbin Unit 731 Sites Protection Regulations and systematised protection of the ruins. In September 2012, the former Unit 731 sites were included on the preparation list of World Heritage Sites in China. The main museum wing was remodelled in 2015, and a new wing and additional preserved ruins in surrounding areas were opened to the public.

The Museum's Current Collection

Based on the former function of each site in Unit 731, there are five different categories within the protected areas: main basic facilities, bacteria and poison gas laboratories, bacterial weapon research and production facilities, experimental animal breeding facilities, and dormitories.

Main Basic Facilities

This includes the central building, facilities supply division and weapons storage, south guard gate, boiler room, railway, water tower, and aviation divisions—totalling seven sites.

The main building, referred to as Building One (一棟) during the war, served as the head office as well as administrative heart of Unit 731. Originally a rectangular two-storey brick and concrete structure, Building One is 170.8 metres long, 13 metres wide, and 15 metres high. From right to left on the first floor were human resources, the duty room, public work division, photography office of the investigation division, office for the head of the investigation division, investigation division general affairs office, warehouse, gendarmerie office, general affairs office, printing room of the investigation division, and the clinic. From right to left on the second floor were rooms for the division and vice-division heads, the planning division, spiritual activities, general affairs, accounting, conference, and artefacts exhibition.

The location of the facilities supply division and weapons storage was referred to as Building Two (二棟) in the old days. This place supplied and housed all the equipment and medical materials. This building was destroyed in the 1970s. Part of the roof was elevated while another part of the building was levelled out. The whole site was remodelled in 2015 (see Fig. 38).

The weapons store kept knives, guns, and ammunition. South guard gate, the only gate out of the original five that remains on the site, served as security checkpoint for entrance to the main building. The boiler room supplied heat and electricity to the main building; only one wall and two chimneys remain. One underground pool for collecting the backwater from the boiler, two remaining walls and thirty-nine heat emission holes still exist. In 2015, the Archaeology Research Center of the Heilongjiang provincial government conducted a comprehensive excavation of the sites of the boiler room and nearby facilities.

The railway built in 1935 connected to Pingfang station and was mainly used to transport staff, experimental animals, and other commodities. The water tower supplied water for the entire complex. The aviator division established in 1938 served field experimentation and biological warfare. This division and the bacteria experimental division conducted many human experiments in the Anda and Chengzigou fields.

These seven places comprised the comparatively well-preserved sites of the basic facilities in Unit 731. They were well-planned and well-equipped with functions that supplied weapons, facilities for experimental use, fuel supply, and field experimentation. They were supported with railways, roads, and aviation facilities that allowed each research centre to enjoy abundant resources and protection. From administration, heat, water, and electricity supplies, transportation to communication, Unit 731 was Japan's efficient core organisation for planning and launching biological warfare.

Bacteria and Poison Gas Laboratories

The major laboratories remaining in the ruins include the Sifanglou (Square Headquarters), the special prison, laboratories for tuberculosis, frostbite and poison gas experiments, and the sites of the poison gas storage room and crematories.

The First Division of Unit 731 for bacteria research focused on bacteria breeding, experiments, and research. Prior to this division, there were a few classes, including plague class, cholera class, typhoid fever class, etc. Unit 731 specially established a poison gas laboratory to conduct experiments on poison gases, to research and produce poison gas. The laboratory used live humans and animals as subjects, and these were ultimately burned in the crematory, a support facility for the bacteria and poison gas laboratory.

Sifanglou, the core area of Unit 731 for human experimentation, was combined with the third, fourth, fifth, and sixth buildings, totalling three stories of 150 metres high and 100 metres wide. Upon the defeat of Japan, Sifanglou was the major facility targeted for destruction by staff, but a large part of the building remained undestroyed at the end of the war. Due to subsequent human activities and natural disasters, however, the relics of the building no longer exist except for its foundation. Sifanglou was bisected by a south–north corridor into east and west wings. Each wing contained a two-storey special prison; the seven-storey west wing imprisoned male '*marutas*' (prisoners). The east wing, also known as the eighth building, kept mainly female *marutas* (see Fig. 40).

The cholera laboratory served for research, bacteria production, and experimentation, while the frostbite laboratory used living prisoners for experiments and production of the drying bacteria for treatment of frostbite (see Fig. 39).

The poison gas laboratory was Unit 731's centre for poison gas experimentation. Test subjects of poison gas were mostly prisoners who had survived bacteria experiments. In order for unit staff to record fatal symptoms and death, the prisoners were confined along with chickens, dogs, mice, and doves. The poison gas storage room was a cylindrical-shaped brick and concrete structure with a curved roof that contained one ground floor and two basement floors. The building was 5.3 metres tall with a diameter of 13 metres.

There were three crematories: the one located north-west of Sifanglou was used to burn corpses and was destroyed by the Unit before the Japanese retreated from Harbin. This site is demolished. Two crematories remain: the Beigang crematory and Beiwadi crematory (see Fig. 41).

These structures made up the core of bacteria and poison gas experimentation of Unit 731, as well as serving as the connecting point for special transportation (of prisoners to be used as subjects) between the Unit and the Kanto Army. A large number of Chinese, Russians, and Koreans were used in experimentation. In the past, scholars believed Unit 731 was responsible for only bacteria research and experiments, and named it '731 bacteria division', which is not completely accurate. In addition to bacteria experiments, the Unit conducted numerous experiments using poison gas. Gas laboratories and storage rooms are evidence of the Unit's activities in frostbite, cholera, typhoid fever, plague, tuberculosis, and anthrax experiments. The three large-scale crematories inside the core area of the headquarters reveal the Unit often used humans for experiments, then destroyed their dead bodies.

Facilities for Research and Creation of Bacterial Weapons

Facilities for bacterial weapon research and creation included an assembly laboratory, weapon class, bombshell factory, and the former experiment field at Chengzigou. The bacteria bombshell factory built and stored bacteria bombs and was managed by the facility supply division. It was a rectangular brick and concrete building with two underground storage rooms. The weapon class aimed to conduct research and build bacteria bombs and other weapons, while focused on research and production of vaccines and serum. It was built in a Chinese courtyard style similar to the Chinese character *Hui* (回).

Serum research took place on the east side of the building, and on the south side were the high-temperature laboratory, sterilisation chamber, and research rooms for the construction of small bacteria bombs. Large weapons such as cars and tanks were stored at the west and north sides. The entire weapons division was destroyed by Unit 731 at the end of the war.

Unit 731's third division conducted research into bacteria pollution, epidemic prevention and water purification and filtration, built ceramic bombshells, and included an earthenware filter pipes building. The factory was located in the Pingxin village at Nangang, Harbin (once called *yangmajiazi*). Five sites of former bombshell factories exist: an office, two kilns, and two chimneys.

The Unit used the Chengzigou experiment field for testing outdoor bacteria and poison gas deployment. It was located 1.5 metres south of Pingle village at Pingxin, Harbin, the historical site of the town of Pingle during the Jin dynasty (1115–1234).

Unit 731 secretly conducted research and construction of bacterial weapons, even though its stated official aim was 'epidemic prevention and water purification'. All these facilities are evidence of experimentation research, construction, storage, and transportation of bacterial weapons.

We have learned from the reliable sources that earthenware bacteria bombs were the most numerous bombs produced by Unit 731. The scale of the factory and the abandoned shells are living evidence that the Unit aimed to carry out biological warfare. Moreover, 'The Thompson Report' recorded the research process of Unit 731 on biological weapons production, including experiments and bomb production methods. The drawing provided by Shirō Ishii, which was mentioned elsewhere, is the model that Unit 731 produced, which might be the collective achievement of the shell factory, weapon class, and other departments.

Experimental Animal Breeding Facilities

In order to maintain a stable and continuous supply of experimental animals, Unit 731 established permanent breeding facilities and separate rooms for ground squirrel, insects, horses, cows, and sheep. Animals kept by Unit 731 included ground squirrel, mice, rabbits, monkeys, horses, cows, sheep, camels, deer, and others used as experimental objects in bacteria and poison gas experiments. Animals served as medium to spread fleas, lice, bedbugs, flies, and mosquitoes. The remaining sites from the experimental animal breeding facilities are animal breeding rooms, ground squirrel breeding room, and insects cultivate room.

Animal breeding rooms kept mice and rabbits. The facility was managed by the Ishii division, headed by Shirō Ishii's older brother, technician Mitsuo Ishii. The ground squirrel breeding room kept ground squirrel, the most commonly used animal by Unit 731. Unit 731 was also called by the name 'Mouse Force' (see Fig. 42).

The insect cultivation room was where Unit 731 kept fleas, lice, bedbugs, flies, and mosquitoes used for bacterial infection. The former site of the cultivate room had south and north wings. The south wing was a single-storey, shaped like the Chinese character '*ao*' (凹). In the middle was another single-storey building, shaped like the

Chinese character '*gong*' (工), and a two-storey building north wing, shaped like the character '*yi*' (一). A few walls remain on the site.

Unit 731 built a few experimental animal breeding facilities and bought a large number of mice. The large-scale facilities and mice were used to produce plague bacteria and plague vaccine for the Japanese troops. The huge quantity of plague bacteria remaining in the former site proved a disaster for Chinese civilians after the Unit retreated and plague broke out in Harbin.

Dormitory

The dormitory of Unit 731, also known as Togo Dormitory, Tougo Village, and Sergeant Building, housed sergeants, army surgeons, soldiers, and their relatives. Currently, thirty-four buildings of dormitory remain on the site in Pingfang area (see Fig. 43).

Unit 731 had the largest residential complex among all other dormitories of the Japanese Army anywhere, which proved that the scale and financial funding of the Unit was also the largest. In addition to a dormitory for families, a dormitory for singles, a dormitory for officers, and facilities that supplied water and heat, the compound also contained a school, post office, hospital, library, sport ground, restaurant, brothel, and the Tougo Shrine. The public facilities such as the library, hospital, sports ground, and post office served as mentally healing spots for the army surgeons, 'experts', and 'experimenters' attempting to help normalise their cruel routine duties.

These former sites of Unit 731 are all listed under the general planning of the city of Harbin as well as the 'Plan for Protection of the Former Sites of Unit 731 of the Japanese Army Invading China' (侵华日军第七三一部队旧址保护规划) announced by Heilongjiang Province in 2014.

Unit 731 Museum

The surrender of Japan and the end of the Second World War on the Eastern Front occurred on 15 August. Unit 731 Museum chose 15 August for its three openings: the first in 1985, the second opening of the new building, south-east of former sites, in 1995, and the renewal of the museum in 2015.

New Building

The new building south-east of the former Unit 731 sites is 24,000 square metres and covers 11,000 square metres of land. Construction started in November 2014. It was designed by the School of Architecture of South China University of Technology with He Jingtang as chief designer. The exhibition was designed by Luode Cultural Engineering Co. Ltd.

As an academic advisor for the exhibition in the new building, I was responsible for designing the layout and content, as well as descriptive writing. When the first draft for the exhibition was confirmed, designers from Japan, Korea, Britain, and Canada were invited to evaluate and comment on the draft. The finalised ideas of the design were 'Simple, Plain, Real, Objective' (see Fig. 44).

Exhibits

Most of the exhibits are genuine artefacts from the former Unit 731 sites, including pictures, graphs, maps, models, videos, and touchable screens. The setting is based on traditional historical museum design incorporating modern exhibition methods. The exhibition display texts are supported by the objects, historical materials, and oral narrative that reveal the facts of Japanese biological warfare as it took place in Harbin.

The new museum is 4,500 square metres, comprising six sections: Japan's biological warfare against China; Unit 731 as the headquarters of the biological warfare; human experimentation; creation of biological weapons; implementation of biological warfare; and the destruction of evidence and post-war trial. These sections uncover and display the historical truth, the cruelty of the Imperial Japanese Army in biological warfare, in order to relate war crimes and war responsibilities of Japan to the public and to emphasise our mission: 'remember the history, never forget the past, love peace and build the future'.

The new building houses more than 10,000 artefacts from the ruins, more than half of them directly related to Unit 731. The building utilises historical sources from China, the US, and Japan, especially the documents about the 'special transfer' available only in China, records of commands with regard to biological warfare existing in Japan, and the recently declassified confidential documents about Unit 731 made public by the US. The entire exhibition is a combination of academic research and common exhibition that used an abundance of photographic, graphic, and simulated scenes to recreate the actual sites that allow visitors to explore history by stepping inside the sites.

The Meaning and Values of Sites Protection

Since war's end in 1945, remaining ruins can reveal the truth of history. Along with city development, it is essential to re-evaluate the historical and social values of the historical sites and learn the historical messages that the ruins bring to the present. To protect and make use of the remaining sites of Unit 731 will therefore be invaluable to facilitate patriotic education and to highlight the important message of peace and the hatred of war.

In summation, the protection of former Unit 731 sites can be seen as generating the following meanings and values:

1. The former sites display invaluable messages and serve as evidence of war crimes. These remaining sites are huge, facilitating inhuman activities ranging from

human experimentation to animal and insect breeding. The Japanese scientists and technicians conducted research on bacteria weapons by murdering thousands of living '*marutas*' from China, Korea, Russia, and the United States. It was the place where Unit 731 created, stored, and distributed the biochemical weapons of massive destruction that could wipe out the entire human race. All cruel and gruesome functions of Unit 731 were well-planned and well-equipped.

2. The former sites are well-preserved. Today, viewers are able to comprehend the original structure and function of the Unit 731 compound. The natural erosion of the sites is now under control. As such, we are able to study and understand the complex organisation and activities within this highly restricted and mysterious campus.

3. Unit 731 is an integrated zone that combined experimental research, armament production and storage, outdoor experimental fields, animal breeding, and living areas. The effective design of the zone allowed Unit 731 to become the headquarters for planning, organising, and execution of biological warfare for Japan, making it also the largest biological weapons production field in human history.

4. The former sites of Unit 731 are incontrovertible evidence that biological warfare was the main purpose of the Unit. By secretly produced bacteria weapons and poison gases, and supported by frostbite experiments and bacterial infection and prevention, Unit 731 was an inhumane and unethical special division during the Second World War.

5. Unit 731's former sites served as the living evidence of the Japanese's war crimes in China. Many of the Chinese and foreigners who fought against Japan, together with many innocent civilians, lost their lives in these sites. These sites will remain important artefacts for scholars to conduct research on Japanese war crimes.

6. The former sites of Unit 731 are an important educational base to teach the world the importance of peace. This is a memorial site for the Anti-Fascist War worldwide. Similar to Auschwitz concentration camp in Poland and Hiroshima Peace Memorial in Japan, Unit 731's sites are there to remind the world of the important message of 'No more war but peace'.

East and West,
Harbin to Auschwitz

Harbin, a city in north-east China, is cold for more than six months a year. The weather has shaped people who are bold, forthright, passionate, and enthusiastic. This is a city that matured and expanded in the twentieth century when Russia began building the Far East Railway there, starting a new page in global history.

Even Chinese find its pronunciation odd, and those arriving in Harbin often ask its meaning: the name is from the Manchu language used by Manchu residents there since the seventeenth century, which literally means a place for drying fish nets. The city adjoins the Songhua River, which is famous for fishing, and fishermen dry their nets nearby.

In addition to Chinese, a large number of Russians, Japanese, and Jews were residing in Harbin between 1900 and 1931. The often-frozen city enjoyed foreign influences and was tolerant and open. On 18 September 1931, Japan began its invasion of China with the Mukden Incident (also known as 'The 918 Incident'). Tragedy was set in motion on 5 February 1932 with the occupation of Harbin by the Japanese military. Then, in August 1933, the Japanese Army created Unit 731, whose terrible and inhumane acts became an indelible nightmare for people of Harbin. Today, on 18 September every year, the air defence alarm sounds three times to memorialise the disaster and to remind people who are living in peace that their beloved city was once filled with tears and pain.

What befell Harbin has left marked effects on the past, present, and future of the city. In 1905, the Qing government set up the '*Binjiang Guandao Yamen*' ('administrative office at Binjiang border') at Harbin. After the collapse of Qing autonomy, the *Beiyang* government and later the local warlords became its official administrators. Russia, which was building the Far East Railway through Harbin, became involved in the city's political and economic activities as well. Japanese involvement in Harbin also dates to the Russo-Japanese War (1904–1905).

Harbin expanded and developed under this tense situation: the city was filled with colonial and anti-colonial sentiments and tension between powers increased continually with changing political circumstances. Although it is little-known by the public, Harbin was home to a large number of Jews in the first half of the twentieth century.

The Historical Connection between Jews and Harbin

People without a country, Jewish people have survived through their strong will as an independent nation for millennia. In the twentieth century, many settled along the Jordan River on the Arabian Peninsula and established the homeland of Israel. From the end of the nineteenth century to the beginning of the twentieth century, a large number arrived at Harbin, where discrimination, rejection, and persecution were rare—it was a land where they were able to use their talents and skills.

In 1899, S. I. Bertsel, the first Jewish settler in Harbin, was followed by others seeking a better place to live. As conditions worsened for Jews in the larger world, especially after the defeat of Russia in the Russo-Japanese War, a group of enlisted Jews deserted from the Russian troops and settled in Harbin. As the immigrants enjoyed recovery, their businesses benefited Harbin's culture, economy, and civic development in many ways, repositioning the Chinese city with a foreign colour. Today, many Jewish historical sites have been preserved in Harbin including a synagogue, Jewish secondary schools, hospitals, and a cemetery.

Harbin's resident Jews were actively involved in business activities in the first half of the twentieth century. Their rapid economic development became their golden age, as from 1900 to 1920, Harbin was internationalised. To become an international city requires a strong economy, rising population, an advantageous regional location, and mature development in city, culture, and facilities. Jews in Harbin established banks, enterprises, trading companies, and industrial factories beneficial to the city. They also introduced social and natural sciences, culture, and art from Europe. Harbin was thus the most permanent city in China to learn about and apply western culture to local growth.

When the Japanese invaded Harbin in 1932, they expelled Jews from the city. However, the Japanese sought to utilise talents and attract investment by Jewish residents, so the Japanese Manchukuo started The Fugu Plan, proposing that Jews be encouraged to settle in Manchukuo to develop and establish 'the New Order in Greater East Asia'. In 1940, when Japan allied with Germany, Gestapo Col. Josef Albert Meisinger visited China and demanded the expulsion of Jewish people from China with the help of the Japanese Army. The Japanese plan to build a Jewish independent country in Northeast China had no chance to succeed. What happened to the Jews on the European continent at the same period?

To Auschwitz

Long before I heard of Unit 731, I knew Germany killed Jews and others in the Holocaust. I first learned about Auschwitz and other death camps in high school when I watched the film *Schindler's List* directed by Steven Spielberg. The movie was a great shock to me.

Years later, on a winter night alone in Harbin, I watched *Schindler's List* again. I learned about the fear and pain of people facing death, the cruel and inhuman behaviour of man, as well as the mixture of kind-heartedness and evil. I believe 'great' is inadequate to describe Oskar Schindler. As a Nazi party member, arms trader, public speaker, and expert in social skills, he saved more than 1,100 lives.

When I finished the movie at 1 a.m., I was thinking as to whether there had been a man who stepped out from Unit 731 and saved the victims (*marutas*), especially the children—it would have been so great, so meaningful. My wish did not happen historically. History only shows endless torture and death: no survivors and no last words from the victims.

I cannot sleep when this history crosses my mind. I feel hopeless and breathless. Only pain remains in the room. Films and reading about Germany's death camps were inadequate for me to understand them, the mentality of their leaders, and their commonality with what took place in China under the Japanese. My first visit in summer 2012 to the concentration camp and museum in Auschwitz, Poland, was deeply disturbing.

Concentration Camp

The German Army constructed their first concentration camp in April 1940. To process a growing population of prisoners there, they then built No. 2 and No. 3 camps at the site. These first three camps are now 'Former Nazi German Auschwitz-Birkenau Concentration Camps', and the first two are open to public visitors. Citizens of more than thirty countries were interned in the camps, including Hungarians, Poles, Gypsies, Russians, and one Chinese, who remains only a number—181292—without further information.

On 27 January 1945, the Russian Red Army liberated Auschwitz-Birkenau and set more than 7,000 survivors (including more than 130 children) free. More than 1.5 million perished in the camps. The Russian Red Army found 7.7 tons of hair and personal belongings from victims, including suitcases, shoes, and glasses.

Angel of Death: Josef Mengele

In Auschwitz, SS Capt. Dr Josef Mengele, nicknamed the 'Angel of Death', carried out human experimentation and genetic experiments as terrible as the crimes Unit 731 committed in China. In his book *Deciphering the History of Japanese War Atrocities: The Story of Doctor and General Shiro Ishii*, American scholar Kenneth Port mentions Josef Mengele: 'Shirō Ishii and the doctors of Unit 731 committed horrors on human subjects that only the Dr Mengele of the world might contemplate. Ishii accomplished what Mengele could only dream about'.[1]

At the end of the Second World War, Josef Mengele was released from a POW camp by falsifying his identity. Wanted for war crimes, he was unable to live freely in Germany, so he escaped to South America and evaded trial. With the help of Nazi sympathisers, Mengele continually changed his identity to hide from German police and the Mossad (Israeli intelligence) blacklist. He travelled to Brazil, Paraguay, and other places, and eventually died at the age of sixty-nine of a stroke while swimming. Mengele was never able to return to his motherland. In 1972, Mengele wrote in his diary: '*Aber wie ist heute meine Heimat? Und ist sie noch meine Heimat? Wird sie mich nicht als Feind empfangen?*' ('What is my homeland today? Is it still my homeland? Would they not see me as enemy?')

No matter if they were babies or elders, Mengele killed Jews and others in human experimentation without mercy. In this, he and Shirō Ishii have many similarities: the two were both supporters and perpetrators of human experimentation and both escaped international trials for their war crimes.

Shirō Ishii was not pursued by the Soviet Union, the Chinese government, or the Japanese police. His name is unheard by the post-war generation. When the Second World War ended, Shirō Ishii enjoyed privileges with a prestigious job and stable life. Josef Mengele would have envied him had he known of Ishii's tranquil post-war life in Japan.

Preservation of Ruins and Museum

Just before the end of the Second World War, the Nazis set fire to their camps in order to destroy evidence. The wooden floors, doors, and windows burned, but many structures survived the fire.

Documents that survive include lists of roles played by Nazis and victims, lists leaked by the war criminals in some cases. These precious materials became useful trial exhibits to document Nazi crimes as well as historical displays that reveal what took place in the camps.

On 2 July 1947, the historical site of Auschwitz became the Auschwitz-Birkenau Memorial and Museum. Its permanent exhibition halls utilise photos, relics, and historical documents to depict its tragic history. One showcase about 30 metres long contains human hair and shoes from little boys and girls, men and women. Those who died in the camps left only these nameless belongings, as if they were never alive in this world. I dare not to guess what feelings Jews today hold toward Germany and her people. As a Chinese citizen, knowing how my countrymen suffered such similar disaster, I was not able to act like the ordinary visitors touring the concentration camps in a hurry without any emotional reaction.

On 7 December 1970, Chairman of the Federal Republic of Germany Willy Brandt fell to his knees when he visited a monument to the Nazi-era Warsaw Ghetto Uprising. With this gesture, the '*Warschauer Kniefall*', he was awarded the 1971 Nobel Peace Prize for his act of contrition for his countrymen and their crimes. In 1979, UNESCO listed Auschwitz-Birkenau concentration camp as a world heritage site to spread the message 'love peace, no war' to the world. In 1996, German Chancellor Helmut Kohl proclaimed 27 January as International Holocaust Remembrance Day to remind countrymen to never forget their history of Holocaust.

In the same year, the ruins of the US atomic attack on Hiroshima, Japan, were listed as a World Heritage site by UNESCO. Based on UNESCO's criteria that such sites '… be an outstanding example of a type of building, architectural or technological ensemble or landscape which illustrates (a) significant stage(s) in human history', Auschwitz-Birkenau and Hiroshima easily qualify.

In 2012, the historical ruins of Unit 731 in Harbin were included onto the preliminary list from China for submission to the UNESCO. This action came late, in our opinion, but it reflects the desire for peace, freedom, and human rights by Chinese people.

Germany does not forget its history of great contributions to a better world, it also does not ignore mistakes its countrymen made in the past. This allows citizens to study their own history in a critical way from the perspective of human rights and ethics. This is what we consider a civilised country. We do not think it is necessary for a national leader to make a public display in another country, although Willy Brandt's act of sorrow represented, indeed, an apology and deep reflection from his heart. Actions, not words, are more meaningful and convincing.

In today's Japan, meanwhile, some scholars and politicians endeavour to cover the truth and fabricate history to deceive the public. The silent members of Unit 731 are the opposite of the honourable Germans who are brave enough to admit their errors. Some forty years after Brandt's gesture, on 12 May 2013, Japan's Prime Minister Shinzō Abe boarded a trainer jet numbered '731' in Matsushima city at Miyagi Prefecture. He smiled and posed with thumbs up for a photo. Released by Japanese media, this image drew great international attention. Abe was undoubtedly aware of the sensitive nature of the number on the jet. The incident reflects the Abe administration's attitude of not admitting, not reflecting, and not apologising for Imperial Japan's war crimes. We concur with the comment from South Korea's *Joong Ang Daily* on the incident: 'Abe's behaviour is unbelievable. Imagine if the leader of Germany rides on a trainer jet in a Nazi uniform…'

Remembering Auschwitz

I left Auschwitz through the gate inscribed with '*Arbeit Macht Frei*' ('Work Sets You Free'), realising the irony of the word '*frei*' ('freedom') at any concentration or extermination camp. The two words have no connection. History, however, linked them together: '*frei*' was taken away and '*Arbeit*' was a pretext for massacre.

I could not calm myself as I rode back to Krakow that rainy autumn afternoon. I thought of the buildings, and how terror saturated their bricks. I had walked floors once bathed in blood and crime. I could not recall the camp objectively.

On the soil of Auschwitz, we are no longer scholars or visitors, but human beings who look at history with mercy and conscience. We learn about the conflicts between people and nations. Such remaining sites as these camps test the conscience of human beings. They evoke the history of disaster and the countless lives of men and women, young and old, taken without reason.

It is a history that can never be accepted: Europeans created much of civilisation from the Renaissance to the Industrial Revolution and introduced the concepts of basic human rights, freedom, and equality. How and why did some of Europe turn to brutality and inhumane treatment of other nations, acts that provoked war and rewrote the history of their world with blood? Following the end of the Second World War, some Germans chose not to marry or have children, others refused medical treatment as a way to punish themselves and their countrymen who violated world peace on such a massive scale.

I have studied books, official documents, photos, and documentaries that reveal the facts about the Japanese invasion of China. I have met Japanese veterans who participated in massacres in China, and Chinese victims who suffered from the disaster. I could not ignore the emotional damage to my own nation, and I started recording this history to share with people around me, as well as through the internet, in order to reveal this utterly unmitigated evil.

As for those who are still covering this up, those who publish falsified history textbooks, what do they think about the real history?

While I personally do not have a religion or believe in an afterlife, I do believe in and hope for justice. I feel the perpetrators—in this case, the Japanese government, the military, and supporters—were unable to accept justifiable trial and punishment.

After wartime bloodshed, peace and world order are restored, but the cycle of war and peace will begin again. Must we suffer this endlessly?

As a student, I often contemplated the value of life, faith, and desire. As we learn more history of the Second World War and walk through these historical sites, horrific scenes make us doubt the truth of our stated beliefs about the value of life. When I visited Germany for fieldwork on this book, I saw high-tech development in industrial technology and sophisticated social management. These seem vastly distant from the war history of that country.

The world has bought us illusions in order to enable us to accept and live in the present. We try to forget war, death, lies, and conflict. When one tries to trace the past, the facts discourage us from seeking the truth. I think of the destiny of human beings: were the Jews alive during the Second World War born to face death and danger? From this point of view, I wonder what the Japanese Army surgeons felt when they took scalpels to the bodies of hopeless Chinese, Russians, and Koreans on the operating table.

Is all this not worthy of serious investigation? Is nationality defining our destiny? The instigators of war steal land, utilise military power to occupy weaker nations, kill the innocent, and shatter order. Today, similar situations take place throughout the world, there is little sign of true world peace. The world is the same, as the Bible says: 'The thing that hath been, it is that which shall be; and that which is done is that which shall be done: and there is no new thing under the sun'.[2]

Why Do We Record History?

I was once asked, 'As a member of a younger generation who did not suffer from war and was born after the opening of China, why do you study Chinese history, especially focusing on the most humiliating era?' I told them my reasons.

Initially, I studied this specific aspect of Chinese history because of my job. As I learned through copious research, however, I uncovered cruelty beyond human imagining. All these acts happened in the land we Chinese are living in, and unfortunately, there are far too many people in China and the rest of the world who have not heard this history.

There is a Chinese saying: 'When there are adequate stores, they will know decorum; when the people have enough of food and clothing, they will know honour'. We are living in a materialistic world, but we forget to learn about our past, and there is an urgent need to reveal it to people, such as those whose only aim is making a fortune.

I used to think the current world situation might be changed. India's statesman Gandhi said, 'You must be the change you want to see in the world,' so I started with myself, and I began to record this largely untold history. Every time I met with family members of the victims of Unit 731, I had a strong urge to tell the world what happened in Unit 731. Through our conversations, I gathered better understanding of how history has treated these families and of their pain. They became the driving force for me to carry on my investigation.

Is history important? I am asked why history matters, why historical research on Unit 731 is still essential. I replied, explained, and argued with those who want to leave it in the past, those who said the surviving sites are sufficient.

One Japanese person I interviewed told me: 'If you [the Chinese] all forget the history, how can you assume we [the Japanese] will remember?' All historical events, good and bad, are worth recording and are important to a country and to a nation state. These are all part of our collective experience. As professional researchers, we have the responsibility to document history, reveal the truth to the public, and tell the world what exactly has taken place. Only through recording history can we tell both Chinese and foreigners the causes for each event, and in preserving historical sites, we express their value. Being objective and conducting reliable historical research are the key to the world's respect.

Assessing Student Recognition of Unit 731 and Auschwitz

The Research Society for the Fifteen Years' War and the Japanese Medical Science and Service collected data from surveys on 10 October 2010 to assess recognition of Unit 731 and Auschwitz among Japanese undergraduate and graduate medical students. The survey found the following that 68 per cent of students know about Auschwitz; 27 per cent of them have heard of it; 5 per cent of them did not know what Auschwitz is; 17

per cent knew about Unit 731; 21 per cent of them have heard the name; and 62 per cent knew nothing about Unit 731.

Regarding Unit 731, the survey posed the question: do you think the medical field should attest to their roles and apologise? The results show that 69 per cent of students thought the medical field should attest and apologise in public; 25 per cent were unsure if this is necessary; and 6 per cent of them rejected the suggestion.

When asked if it affects current issues, 75 per cent of the students agreed, 6 per cent of them disagreed, while 19 per cent were unsure.

In general, recognition of the history of Unit 731 among medical students in Japan is low. The fact that 62 per cent of them have no knowledge of Unit 731 cannot compare with the high recognition of Auschwitz among European students. Since the surveys were conducted in Tokyo among presumably well-educated subjects, recognition of Unit 731 might be even lower in other prefectures in Japan. As Unit 731 has seldom appears in Japanese history textbooks, it may be forgotten as time goes by.

Fortunately, this survey revealed a positive result as well: more than half of those surveyed agreed that official attestations and apologies should be made by the Japanese medical field, reflecting that the public now understands the relationship between war crimes and the responsibility of the medical field, as well as the interrelated influence of international affairs.

Many Japanese scholars told me more than 99 per cent of Japanese have never heard of Unit 731. Despite this, Japanese author Seiichi Morimura's work *Akuma no Housyoku* (悪魔の飽食 *The Devil's Gluttony*) published in 1981 has been reprinted more than fifty times and sold over 3 million copies. As of today, the population of Japan exceeds 126 million, meaning 2.3 per cent of the population have heard of Unit 731. Thus, Morimura made a great contribution to improve low recognition of Unit 731 in Japan.

With the outbreak of the Korean War, the US cooperated with its ally Japan, which was nicknamed the 'Aircraft carrier that never sinks', to fight Communism. Some of the dried plasma used in the war was supplied by the 'Green Cross', a pharmaceutical corporation established by Ryoichi Naitō of the former Unit 731. Japan supplied materials to the Korean front without directly supplying manpower, making huge profits and enabling its economy to recover at high speed. The development of Japan's electrical, motor, and light industries were vigorous enough that Japan hosted its first Olympic Games in 1964, just nineteen years after its surrender.

As Chinese, we are happy to witness our close neighbour's economy, culture, society, and the well-being of its people thriving. Although Japan has enjoyed phenomenal development to the degree its history in the Second World War and its invasion of China are deliberately forgotten by many of its people, we must stay alert.

About thirty Japanese Prime Ministers have been in office since the end of the Second World War. Beginning with Yoshida Shigeru in 1951, many of them have visited the Yasukuni Shrine. Prior to the 1970s, Prime Ministers visited in private and avoided 15 August (the date of Japan's surrender). Miki Takeo was the first to visit Yasukuni

Shrine on that date and did so privately. In 1982, Prime Minister Fukuda Yasuo visited it as the Chief Cabinet Secretary of Japan. That year, Japan changed 15 August from 'Memorial Day for the end of the war' to 'Day for mourning war dead and praying for peace'.

Between 2001 and 2006, Prime Minister Jinichiro Koizumi visited Yasukuni Shrine six years consecutively, while current Prime Minister Shinzō Abe visited in 2013. Both China and South Korea expressed their disappointment and anger toward the visits of Yasukuni Shrine by Japanese officials, but their protests failed to affect the attitude of Japanese government and the officials.

Yasukuni Shrine, a religious site before the war, is now a national symbol of Japanese militarism whose supporters encourage worship of the emperor system of Japan and devote themselves to serve Japan's national needs, including war. Even though the shrine has become an independent religious corporation in post-war Japan, it still serves as a spiritual representation of former Japanese militarism.

Why does Yasukuni Shrine matter to China and Korea? On 4 November 2015, I visited Yasukuni Shrine and its Yūshūkan (遊就館), a Japanese military and war museum, and viewed the exhibition '70th Year After the Great East Asia War'. I saw only glorified descriptions of the Great East Asia War and the loyalty of Japanese soldiers to the Emperor of Japan. Nowhere did the exhibit mention 'invasion', 'regret', or 'aggression'. The museum is a place that 'promotes aggressive war and extension of Japan'. Yasukuni Shrine notes the death of more than 2,460,000 soldiers of Japan, including those involved in aggressive wars by Japan during the Second World War, such as Hideki Tojo, Iwane Matsui, and twelve other class-A war criminals as well as more than 2,000 class-B and class-C criminals. All these dead officials are described as 'inventors' to China and Korea, including the fourteen class-A war criminals sentenced to death or imprisonment at the Tokyo Trial in 1946–1948. They are now honoured in Yasukuni Shrine, and publicly worshiped by Japanese citizens, the premier, and members of the cabinet.

When I visited Yasukini Shrine, I thought of Israel's Mossad, which sent agents to South America to apprehend remaining Nazis. They arrested and kidnaped them, and used Israel's official planes to send them to Israel in secret. Their goal was to see Nazis stand trial and receive punishment for their deeds in the Second World War. How will remaining Nazi members and later generations regard the actions of Mossad? For Israelis and Jews, the Second World War is continuing until justice is served. The Germans chose to accept history with the *Warschauer Kniefall*. Why would Shinzō Abe visit Yasukuni Shrine without fear or shame? What is the meaning of today's geopolitics, with its historical amnesia and willingness to compromise with distortions, for the victimised countries by Imperial Japan such as Korea, China, Great Britain, the Netherlands, Malaysia, the Philippines, Indonesia, Singapore, Vietnam, Myanmar, the United States, and other nations and their citizens?

I am not pessimistic towards the future, however. There are numerous lawsuits within and outside Japan against the Japanese government and corporations for the war crimes committed by Imperial Japan during the Second World War. They demand the Japanese government and corporations for apology and atonement for the war crimes with regard to the Nanjing Massacre, Military Sexual Slavery ('Comfort Women') System, Forced Labour System, Inhumane Treatment of POWs, or Biochemical Warfare represented by Unit 731. Some of the cases have ended in favour of the plaintiffs in the courts of law. Meanwhile, the Japanese parents have organised the nationwide society, *Kotomo to Kyokasho Zenkoku Netto 21* (Nationwide Network for Children and Textbooks in the 21st Century), to serve as a watchdog to stop textbook revision by the Japanese government. I understand that even Japanese parents living outside Japan have joined the society and subscribed to its newsletter.

I am particularly encouraged in my work in the last few years, thanks to the help and guidance from Professor Yue-him Tam, the academic advisor to our International Center for the Study of Unit 731 and the Museum of War Crimes by Unit 731 of the Imperial Japanese Army in Harbin. A senior historian of Japanese history and Sino-Japanese relations, Professor Tam has been conducting research and teaching a course at his college for years, focusing on the major war crimes and atrocities committed by Imperial Japan, including the biochemical warfare and Unit 731. I consulted him whenever I ran into problems in my research for this book. He was indispensable to facilitate our field work at the US National Archives and Records Administration and the Library of Congress in Washington, DC. He is indeed the author of the English version of this book with his insights that are absent in the Chinese version. I felt honoured and gratified when Professor Tam accepted my invitation to work on this book as co-author, for our research and messages could now reach the minds and hearts in the wider world.

Events Timeline

17 June 1925
Protocol for the Prohibition of the Use in War of Asphyxiating, Poisonous or other Gases, and of Bacteriological Methods of Warfare signed in Geneva, Switzerland

June 1927
Shirō Ishii receives Doctor of Medicine degree from Kyoto Imperial University, Japan

April 1928–April 1930
Shirō Ishii conducts field research in Europe and America on biochemical warfare

1932
Shirō Ishii promoted to army surgeon lieutenant-commander

5 July 1932
Japan Ministry of War permits the Army Medical School to set up Bacteria Research Center with Shirō Ishii as key member of the team researching biochemical weapons

8 December 1932
The Ministry of War of Japan approves an investment of ￥ 208,989 on the expansion of Disease Prevention Research Center in the Army Medical School

April 1933
Bacteria Research Center set up in the temporary shelter for sick horses of the Kanto Army, marking 100th Division of the Kanto Army preparations for biochemical warfare

August 1933
The Disease Prevention Center of the Ministry of War of Japan secretly moves to Xuanhua Street in Harbin. Bacteria Experiment Center established in Beiyinhe of Wuchang city. Often known as the Kamo Unit and the Ishii Unit, the pre-cursor of Unit 731

23 September 1934
Large-scale escape from Beiyinhe Bacteria Experiment Center organised by Northeast Anti-Japanese United Army reveals the existence of human experimentation

1 August 1935
Shirō Ishii promoted to army surgeon lieutenant-colonel

1936
The Kamo Unit begins surveying Pingfang area for construction of large-scale headquarters for biochemical warfare

25 June 1936
The Epidemic Prevention department of the Kanto Army formed on the official establishment date for Unit 731

1937
Kamo Unit begins invention of bacteria bombs

30 June 1938
Kanto Army headquarters announce order no. 1539 'Regarding creation of Special Military Zone around Pingfang' of 120 square kilometres including Pingfang , Japanese Air Force Unit 8372, Unit 731, and other areas. Residents are forced to move out or restricted

1939
Basic facilities and laboratories of Pingfang Special Military Zone completed. Kamo Unit moves into the Special Military Zone, its former site now used by the Third Division

18 April 1939
Nanjing Rong Unit 1644 established
Guangzhou Bo Unit 8604 established

7 July 1939
Headquarters of Kanto Army announce command no. 78 Mobilising Unit 731 for the battles of Khalkhin Gol in Hailar district. Initial use of biochemical warfare by Unit 731 including deploying cholera, typhoid fever, and shigella to pollute river water

23 March 1940
The 'Northern China Epidemic Prevention and Water Purification Department' formed, also known as the Beijing 'A' Unit no. 1855

29 April 1940
Kamo Unit Epidemic Prevention and Water Purification Department and the Fourteenth Division of Army Surgeons publish 'Guidelines for All Epidemic Prevention and Water Purification Departments' rules of general operation, arrangement, duties, and mission

June–November 1940
Unit 731 conducts experiments on plague prevention and field experiments in Changchun and Nongan County

25 July 1940
Kanto Army headquarters issue command no. 659, and its Expeditionary Army Group begins transport of materials for biochemical warfare to Unit 731

26 July 1940
Kanto Expeditionary Army Group announces command no. 178: Harbin, Shenyang, and Jinzhou start transporting materials to Unit 731

1 August 1940
Kanto Epidemic Prevention renamed Kanto Epidemic Prevention and Water Purification Department

4 October 1940
Japanese Army starts biochemical warfare in Quzhou, Zhejiang by air drops of bacteria-infected siphonaptera, wheat, yellow beans, cloth, cotton, and other materials. Plague spreads widely in Quzhou, Zhejang

22 October 1940
Japanese Army launches biochemical warfare in Ningbo, Zhejiang by dropping bacteria-infected siphonaptera, wheat, flour, and other materials by air. Plague spreads in Ningbo, Zhejiang

27–28 October 1940
Japanese Army starts biochemical warfare in Jinhua, Zhejiang, plague spreads in Jinhua and Yiwu, Zhejiang

2 December 1940
Kanto Army Commander Yoshijirō Umezu gives approval for the Kanto Epidemic Prevention and Water Purification Department to set up sub-branches at Hailar, Sunwu, Linkou, and Mudanjijang

1941
Kamo Unit renamed Manchuria Unit 731, Wakamatsu Unit renamed Manchuria Unit 100, Mudanjijang Unit becomes Manchuria Unit 643, Linkou Unit becomes Manchuria Unit 162, Sunwu changes to Manchuria Unit 763, and Hailar renamed Manchuria Unit 543

March 1941
Shirō Ishii promoted to army surgeon major-general

July 1941
Kanto Army carries out large-scale military exercises with 700,000 soldiers in Manchuria

4 November 1941
Japanese Army initiates biochemical warfare in Changde, Huana by aerial drops of bacteria-infected 36 grams of siphonaptera, cloth, beans, wheat, grain, cotton, and other material. Plague breaks out in Changde, Hunan

5 May 1942
Japanese Southern Area Army Unit 9420 set up in Singapore

June–August 1942
Japanese Army drops cholera, typhoid fever, and shigella bacteria by plane on Jinhua and Lanxi, Zhejiang, causing large number of Chinese civilian fatalities

1 August 1942
Shirō Ishii relocates to Northern Area Army as division head of Army Surgeon in the First Division. Masaji Kitano appointed Second Division head of Unit 731

August 1942
Japanese Army places cholera, typhoid fever, and shigella bacteria in wells, river water, and food in Yushan County, Jiangxi. Large numbers of Chinese villagers are reported dead

February 1943
Baitabao event occurs. Mukden Military Police Generals Zhoa Zongbo, Shi Shunchen, and Cui Bingzhang sent to Unit 731

15 February 1943
Kanto Army headquarters announce command no. 98 sending Unit 731 to Shenyang to start 'disease prevention' on British and American POWs

12 March 1943
Kanto Army headquarters announce command no. 120 'About Ultimatum of Special Transportation' setting regulations of special transportation

October 1943
Dalian Heishijiao event: Dalian Military Police Generals Yaoxuan Wang, Xuenian Wang , Zhongshan Li, and Delong Shen specially transported to Unit 731

1 January 1945
Unit 731 announces 'About Remaining behind List of Kanto Epidemic Prevention and Water Purification Department'

1 March 1945
Shirō Ishii becomes division head of Unit 731 again and is promoted to army surgeon lieutenant-general. Masaji Kitano relocates to Shanghai as the division head of Army Surgeons in 'Chinese Expeditionary Army (Shanghai) Thirteenth Army'

9–14 August 1945
Unit 731 destroys evidence of biochemical warfare and human experimentation, bombs headquarters, and sub-branch buildings and facilities

15 August 1945
Japan announces unconditional surrender

9 September 9 1945
Japan signs the instrument of surrender to China in Nanjing

September–October 1945
Lt-Col. Murray Sanders investigates Japanese biochemical warfare and finishes his report 'Investigation Report on Japan Science Information'

February 1946
US investigator Lt-Col. Murray Sanders interrogates core members of Unit 731, including Shirō Ishii, Masaji Kitano, Kiyoshi Oda, and Naitō Ryoichi. US Army investigator Thompson finishes his 'Report of Japanese Biochemical Warfare Research and Preparation'

25–29 December 1949
Soviet Union establishes military court at Khabarovsk and tries twelve Japanese war criminals involved in biochemical warfare. The Khabarovsk Trials official record is published in *Materials on the Trial of Former Servicemen of the Japanese Army Charged with Manufacturing and Employing Bacteriological Weapons*. The book is translated into Chinese, English, German, Japanese, Korean, and other languages

June–July 1956
The People's Republic of China Supreme People's Court Special Military Court puts forty-five Japanese war criminals on trial at Shenyang and Taiyuan, including the head of Linkou Division, Sakakibara Hideo

15 November 1957
Former member of Unit 731 Kaneda Yasushi and others start Unit 731 Companion Club '*Fusatomo Kai*' (房友会) and publish international magazine *Fusatomo*

1958
Former members of Unit 731 establish '*Seikon Tō*' (精魂塔) at Tama Cemetery, Tokyo. They also set up the Companion Club '*Seikon Kai*' (精魂会)

9 October 1959
Shirō Ishii dies in Tokyo due to illness

19 July–3 October 1981
Japanese writer Seiichi Morimura publishes *The Devil's Gluttony* in *Akahata* (赤旗)

October 1981
American journalist John William Powell publishes 'A Hidden Chapter in History' in the Bulletin of Atomic Scientists revealing covert deal between Japan and the US

November 1981
The Devil's Gluttony by Seiichi Morimura is published, revealing Japanese Army biochemical warfare and human experimentation. Translated into Chinese, English, Russian, and other languages, it receives huge international response

1 December 1982
The Cultural and Artefact Management Office of Pingfang area in Harbin was established, which offers protection to the sites of Unit 371

1983
Site of Unit 731 registered as a Heilongjiang's major historical and cultural site protected at the provincial level

1984
The Japan Ministry of Education, Science and Culture deletes mentions of Unit 731 in textbooks

13 August 1985
British independent television company broadcasts a documentary titled *Unit 731: Did the Emperor Know?*

15 August 1985
The Museum of War Crime Evidence by Japanese Army Unit 731 officially opens to public

1988
The film *Men Behind the Sun* shows in movie theatres

July 1989
Human bones discovered on site of the Japanese Army Hospital. Research Group on Human Bones Found in Army Hospital formed in September

September 1989
'Selected Archival Documents on the Invasion of China by the Japanese Imperialists:
   Bacteriological and Poison Gas Warfare' published by State Archives Administration

December 1993
Yoshimi Yoshiaki publishes the hand-written 'Imoto Diary' in *Asahi Shimbun* newspaper

February 1995
Organisation for the Investigation of Japan's Leftover Biochemical Weapons created by Japanese
   grassroots citizens in Japan.

31 July 1995
Heilongjiang Provincial Academy of Social Science and Japan-China Friendship Association
   organise seminar 'Anti-aggression, Maintain Peace' in Harbin. Exhibition tour of Unit 731 starts
   in Japan

15 August 1995
New wing of the Museum of War Crime Evidence by Japanese Army Unit 731 officially opens to
   the public

December 1995
Grassroots organisation in China brings criminal charges against the Japanese government on
   behalf of victims of Japanese biochemical warfare. Members of the Japan Federation of Bar
   Associations including Tsuchiya Kouken and Ichise Keiichirou arrive in Zhejiang, Hunan,
   and other places to investigate and collect evidence for use in legal action against Japanese
   government

October 1997
Chengmin Jin discovers records of 'Special Transfer' on in Heilongjiang Provincial Archives

2 August 1999
The Heilongjiang Provincial Government holds press conference to disclose the records of 'Special
   Transfer'

December 1999
'Research Organisation of Unit 731 Site to be registered on UNESCO World Heritage Site'
   established by a Japanese grassroots group. Unit 731 and poison gas exhibits combined into one,
   renamed ABC Planning Commission (referring to atomic, biological, chemical)

July 2000
Harbin Academy of Social Science and Harbin TV visit Japan to conduct interviews with more
   than twenty former members of Unit 731

28 April 2001
Harbin Academy of Social Science sets up Unit 731 Research Center conducting research and
   exchange on Unit 731

6 September 2001
Jilin Provincial Archives organises press conference to announce discovery of records of 'Special
   Transfer'

18 September 2001
Hunan University of Arts and Science establishes research centre to investigate Japanese bacterial
    warfare

October–November 2001
Leading Team on Protection and Development of Unit 731 Site and the *Harbin Daily* visit Japan for
    second round of field investigation

27 August 2002
Tokyo District Court of Japan concludes the Japanese Army used bacterial warfare on Chinese
    civilians, but refuses to pay compensation to Chinese victims affected by Japanese bacterial warfare

7–9 December 2002
Hunan University of Arts and Science holds 'International Academic Conference of War Crimes
    on Bacterial Warfare'

3 September 2005
Harbin Academy of Social Science holds first international academic conference on Japanese
    bacterial and poison gas warfare at Harbin

2006
Unit 731 site listed as a Major Historical and Cultural Site Protected at the National Level

18 October 2006
Harbin Academy of Social Science cooperates with Korea Stele Forest and Korea Chungcheong
    University for second international academic conference on war crimes of Unit 731 at
    Cheongju, Korea

18–19 November 2006
Hunan College of Arts and Science and the Global Alliance for Preserving the History of WWII
    in Asia hold 'International Academic Conference on Japanese Bacterial Warfare' at Changde,
    Hunan

4–5 September 2007
Harbin Academy of Social Science and Defense University of Mongolia hold 'Lessons from History
    and Contemporary Society–Biochemical and Bacterial Weapons of WWII' in Ulaanbaatar,
    Mongolia

July 2008
Heilongjiang Broadcasting Television films and broadcasts the documentary *Immortal Memory*

18 September 2008
Harbin Academy of Social Science and the Museum of War Crime Evidence by Japanese Army
    Unit 731 hold fourth international academic conference on Unit 731 war crimes at Harbin

2010
Heilongjiang Broadcasting Television films the documentary *Japanese Bacterial Warfare* (episodes
    1–8) and broadcasts on China Central Television (CCTV)

October 2011
A team of researchers from the Harbin Academy of Social Sciences conducted research at the
    National Archives and Records Administration and the Library of Congress in Washington,

DC, where they copied over 20,000 pages of newly declassified confidential documents pertaining to Unit 731. The team was invited to conduct seminars on Unit 731 and biochemical warfare by Imperial Japan at Washington, DC, and Macalester College in Minnesota, USA

2012
Site of Unit 731 posted to the reserve list of world heritage sites in China

27 February 2014
Seventh meeting of the 12th Standing Committee of the National People's Congress declares 3 September the anniversary of victories of Anti-Japanese War of the Chinese People and the World Anti-Fascist War, and 13 December as National Memorial Day of the Nanjing Massacre Kenneth L. Port's book, *Deciphering the History of Japanese War Atrocities: The Story of Doctor and General Shiro Ishii* (Durham, NC: Carolina Academic Press, 2014), unfolds the mysteries of life and work of Shirō Ishii, founder of Unit 731 and mastermind of biochemical warfare in Japan.

15 August 2015
Site of Unit 731 and new wing of the Museum of War Crime Evidence by Japanese Army Unit 731 officially opens to public

24 September 2015
Harbin Academy of Social Science and the Museum of War Crime Evidence by Japanese Army Unit 731 hold fifth international academic conference on Unit 731 war crimes in Harbin

Endnotes

Chapter 1

1. United Nations Office for Disarmament Affairs, unoda-web.s3-accelerate.amazonaws.com/wp-content/uploads/assets/WMD/Bio/pdf/Status_Protocol.pdf, accessed on 21 June 2016.
2. United Nations Office for Disarmament Affairs, disarmament.un.org/treaties/t/bwc/text, accessed on 21 June 2016.
3. Ji Xueren ed., *Qinhua Rijun Duqizhan Shiliji* (*Examples of Poisonous Warfare by the Japan's China Expeditionary Army*) (Beijing: Social Sciences Academic Press, 2008), p. 4.
4. Doc Title: ISHII, Dr. Shiro; Location: 290/12/25/04, RG#331, ENTRY#1331, Box1762, National Archives II of USA, Maryland.
5. Doc Title: 441st CIC report on Shiro ISHII; Location; 270/84/16/05, RG#319, ENTRY#184B, Box549, National Archives II of USA, Maryland.
6. A written material, *Guanyu Shijing Budui de Jie Shao* (Introduction to the Ishii Unit), submitted to the US military by Masaji Kitano the Commander of the Unit 731 on 1 April 1947. The document is now preserved at the National Archives II of USA, Maryland. ·
7. The School of Army Surgeon ed., *Rikkun Kuni Gakkō Gojūnen Shi* (*50 Years of History of the School of Army Surgeon*) (Tokyo: Fujishuppan, 1988), p. 184.
8. Miyatake Go, *Shōgun no Igen: Endō Sanrō no Nikki* (*General's Last Words: Diary of Endō Sanrō*) (Tokyo: The Mainichi Newspaper Co., 1986), p. 77.
9. Han Xiao and Xin Peilin, *Rijun Qisanyi Budui Zuieshi* (*Criminal History of the Unit 731 of the Japanese Military*) (Harbin: Heilongjiang People's Publishing House, 1991), pp. 12-13.
10. Document reference no.: C-17, archive of the International Center for Unit 731 Research.
11. *Qianriben Lujun Junren Yinzhunbei he Shiyong Xijun Wuqi Beikongan Shenpan Cailiao* (*Trial Material of the Case that Former Japanese Army Prepared and Used Bacteriological Weapons*), (Moscow: Waiguo Wenshuji Chubanju, 1950), p. 107.
12. *Ibid.*, p. 256.
13. Document no.: S11-10-42, Archive of Research Institute of Self-Defense of Japan, War Ministry.
14. *Ibid.*, Document no.: S1-3-40.
15. *Qianriben Lujun Junren Yinzhunbei he Shiyong Xijun Wuqi Beikongan Shenpan Cailiao* (*Trial Material of the Case that Former Japanese Army Prepared and Used Bacteriological Weapons*), (Moscow: Waiguo Wenshuji Chubanju, 1950), p. 165.
16. Document Reference no.: C-121. Archive of the Exhibition Hall of Evidences of Crime Committed by Unit 731 of the Japanese Imperial Army.
17. *Qianriben Lujun Junren Yinzhunbei he Shiyong Xijun Wuqi Beikongan Shenpan Cailiao* (*Trial Material of the Case that Former Japanese Army Prepared and Used Bacteriological Weapons*), (Moscow: Waiguo Wenshuji Chubanju, 1950), pp. 204-206.

18. Archive of the Relief and Record Divison, Social Welfare and War Victims' Relief Bureau, Ministry of Health, Labour and Welfare, Japan.
19. Document reference no.: B17-3, Archive of the International Center for Unit 731 Research.
20. Video document reference no.: A18-8, Archive of the International Center for Unit 731 Research.

Chapter 2

1. Kenneth L. Port, *Deciphering the History of Japanese War Atrocities: The Story of Doctor and General Shiro Ishii* (Durham, North Carolina: Carolina Academic Press, 2014), p. xii.
2. Doc. Title: 441st CIC report on Shiro ISHII; Location: 270/84/16/05, RG#319, ENTRY#184B, Box 549, National Archives II of USA, Maryland.
3. Kenneth L. Port, *Deciphering the History of Japanese War Atrocities: The Story of Doctor and General Shiro Ishii* (Durham, North Carolina: Carolina Academic Press, 2014), xii, p. 52.
4. Shuli Ji, *Shuyi (Plague)* (Beijing: People's Medical Publishing House Co. Ltd, 2010), p. 2.
5. *Ibid.*
6. Fukiko Aoki, *Shijingsilang ji xijunzhan budui jie mi (The Secrets of Shirō Ishii and Biological Warfare Force)* (Shanghai: Shanghai Translation Publishing House, 2010), p. 360.
7. Iwasaki Jirō, *Bukka no sesō 100nen (100 Years of the situation of commodity prices)*. (Tokyo: Yomimura Shinbum Sha, 1982).
8. *Qianriben lujunjunren yin zhunbei he shiyong xijunwuqi beikongan shenpancailiao (Material of trials for former Japanese Army Soldiers Who Prepared and Used Biological Weapon)* (Moscow: Waiguo wenshuji chubanju, 2005), p. 302.
9. *Ibid.*, p. 397.
10. Hisato Yoshimura, *Memoir of My 77th Birthday,* (Kyoto: Aotian Yinshua Co.,1984).
11. Ichiro Kadowaki, 'Kyoto Medical College and Unit 731 of Japanese Kwantung Army,' *Journal of Research Society for 15 Years War and Japanese Medical Science and Service* 1 (2000): pp. 42-43.
12. Document Reference no.: A-17. Archive of the Exhibition Hall of Evidences of Crime Committed by Unit 731 of the Japanese Imperial Army.
13. Sheldon H. Harris, *Factories of Death: Japanese Biological Warfare, 1932–1945 and The American Cover-up,* (Routlege: 1996), p. 263.
14. Document reference no.: B-2, Archive of the International Center for Unit 731 Research.
15. Document reference no.: E-21, Archive of the International Center for Unit 731 Research.
16. Video document reference no.: B-3, Archive of the International Center for Unit 731 Research.
17. *Ibid.*
18. Sadao Koshi, *Hinomaru ha akai namida ni (Bloody Tears on Hinomaru)* (Japan: Kyoiku Shiryo Shuppankai, 1983), pp. 126-133.
19. Video document reference no.: B-3, Archive of the International Center for Unit 731 Research.

Chapter 3

1. *Qianriben Lujun Junren Yinzhunbei he Shiyong Xijun Wuqi Beikongan Shenpan Cailiao (Trial Material of the Case that Former Japanese Army Prepared and Used Bacteriological Weapons),* (Moscow: Waiguo Wenshuji Chubanju, 1950), pp. 388-389.
2. Association of Returnees from China, *Qinlue: zaihua riben zhanfan de zhengyan (Invasion: Narrative from Japanese Criminals in China)* (China: Xintong Shushe, 2002), pp. 27-28.
3. Sadao Koshi, *Hinomaru wa akai namida ni (Bloody Tears on Hinomaru)* (Japan: Kyoiku Shiryo Shuppankai, 1983), pp. 32-34.

4. Document reference no. E-1, Archive of the International Center for Unit 731 Research.
5. *Ibid.*, Document reference no. F-6.
6. *Ibid.*, Document reference no. F-5.
7. Document Reference no.: E-2. Archive of the Exhibition Hall of Evidences of Crime Committed by Unit 731 of the Japanese Imperial Army.
8. *Ibid.*, Document Reference no.: E-3.

Chapter 4

1. *Qianriben Lujun Junren Yinzhunbei he Shiyong Xijun Wuqi Beikongan Shenpan Cailiao* (*Trial Material of the Case that Former Japanese Army Prepared and Used Bacteriological Weapons*), (Moscow: Waiguo Wenshuji Chubanju, 1950), p. 21.
2. Guo Sumei, *Renxing de Minmie yu Fusu* (*Obliteration and Revival of Human Nature*), read at the *Seminar on Anti-invasion and Peace-keeping* in Harbin in 1995.
3. Jin Chengmin, *Ribenjun Xijunzhan* (*Bacteriological Warfare of the Japanese Military*) (Harbin: Heilongjiang People's Publishing House, 2008), p. 132.
4. Morimura Seiichi, Zu Binghe tran., *Shiren Moku: Riben Guandongjun Xijunzhan Budui de Kongbu Neimu* (*Ogre's Cave: Terrible Inside Story of the Bacteriological Warfare Unit from Japan's Kwantung Army*) (Beijing: Qunzhong Chubanshe, 1984), pp. 65-66.
5. Han Xiao and Xin Peilin, *Rijun Qisanyi Budui Zuieshi* (*Criminal History of Unit 731 of the Japanese Military*) (Harbin: Heilongjiang People's Publishing House, 1991), pp. 118-119.
6. Brief Summary of New Information About Japanese BW Activities; Location: 290/03/19/02, RG#175, ENTRY#67A4900, Box 196, National Archives II of USA.
7. Central Archives ed., *Riben Diguozhuyi Qinhua Dangan Ziliao Xuanbian: Xijunzhan yu Duqizhan* (*Selected Archival Records of the Japanese Imperialist's Invasion of China: Bacteriological Warfare and Poisonous Gas Warfare*) (Beijing: Zhonghua Book, 1989), p. 72.
8. 'Brief Summary of New Information About Japanese BW Activities'; Location: 290/03/19/02, RG#175, ENTRY#67A4900, Box 196, National Archives II of USA.
9. *Naval Aspects of Biological Warfare*; Author: Inglis, RADM Thomas B.; Location: 190/25/17/07, RG#330, ENTRY#199, Box 103, National Archives II of USA.
10. *Report on Japanese Biological Warfare (BW) Activities*; Location: 2910, RG#IWG Ref. Coll, National Archives II of USA.
11. Matsumura Takao and Tanaka Akira ed., *15nen Senso Gokuhi Shiryōshū Dai 29 Shū Nanasanichi Butai Sakusei Shiryō* (Material written by the Unit 731) (Tokyo: Fujishuppan, 1991), pp. 225-281.
12. Study Group of Hygiene Research in Winter, *Gokuhi Chūmōgun Tōki Eisei Kenkyū Seiseki* (Tokyo: Gendai Shokan, 1941), p. 352.
13. *Ibid.*, p. 133.
14. *Ibid.*, pp. 165-166.
15. Miyatake Go, *Shōgun no Igen: Endō Sanrō no Nikki* (*General's Last Words: Diary of Endō Sanrō*) (Tokyo: The Mainichi Newspaper Co., 1986), p. 77.
16. Matsumura Takao and Tanaka Akira ed., *15nen Senso Gokuhi Shiryōshū Dai 29 Shū Nanasanichi Butai Sakusei Shiryō* (Material written by the Unit 731) (Tokyo: Fujishuppan, 1991), pp. 1-42.
17. *Ibid.*
18. Morimura Seiichi, Zu Binghe tran., *Shiren Moku: Riben Guandongjun Xijunzhan Budui de Kongbu Neimu* (*Ogre's Cave: Terrible Inside Story of the Bacteriological Warfare Unit from Japan's Kwantung Army*) (Beijing: Qunzhong Chubanshe, 1984), pp. 108-109.
19. *Ibid.*, p. 109.
20. *War and Medicine*, an exhibition panel brochure prepared by The Research Society for 15 Years' War and Japanese Medical Science and Service, (Japan: Sanhuishe, 2006), p. 1.

21. Shozo Azami, 'The Medical Crime in the Fifteen Years' War and Our Task Today', *Journal of Research Society for 15 years War and Japanese Medical Science and Service*, vol.12, (Japan: Research Society for 15 years War and Japanese Medical Science and Service, 2011), p. 27.

22. *Ibid.*

Chapter 5

1. NA, RG38, BOX2097: A report by Lt-Col. Arvo T. Thompson, V.C, Army Service Forces, Camp Detrick. Maryland. Report on Japanese Biological Warfare(BW) Activities May 31.1946.

2. Doc Title: Bacteriological Warfare; Location: 2910, RG#IWG Ref. Coll., Author: Masuda Tomosada. National Archives II of USA, Maryland.

3. Doc Title: Interrogation of Colonel Enryo HOJO; Location: 270/13/31/05, RG#319, ENTRY#85.

4. Doc Title: 441st CIC Report on Shiro Ishii; Location: 270/84/16/05, RG#319, Entry#184B, Box 549, National Archives II of USA, Maryland.

5. Doc Title: Summary Report on B.W. Investgations; Location: 290/03/19/03, RG#175, ENTRY#67A4900, Box 196, National Archives II of USA, Maryland.

6. *Qianriben Lujun Junren Yinzhunbei he Shiyong Xijun Wuqi Beikongan Shenpan Cailiao* (*Trial Material of the Case that Former Japanese Army Prepared and Used Bacteriological Weapons*), (Moscow: Waiguo Wenshuji Chubanju, 1950), p. 261.

7. *Ibid.*, p. 69.

8. *Ibid.*, p. 61.

9. No. 78 operation order issued by the Kanto Army Command kept at the Japanese National Archives of Official Documents.

10. Central Archives ed., *Riben Diguozhuyi Qinhua Dangan Ziliao Xuanbian: Xijunzhan yu Duqizhan* (*Selected Archival Records of the Japanese Imperialist's Invasion of China: Bacteriological Warfare and Poisonous Gas Warfare*) (Beijing: Zhonghua Book, 1989), pp. 246-247.

11. Chen Wengui, 'Report on plague in Changteh, Human', *Report of the International Scientific Commission for the Investigation of the Facts Concerning Bacterial Warfare in Korea and China*, (Beijing:1952) p. 195.

12. Chen Zhiyuan, Liu Yi, '12 Cases of Oral History Investigation of Victims of Bacteriological Warfare in Changteh', *Journal of Hunan University of Arts and Science*, vol. NO. 2006-03-10, (Changteh: Hunan University of Arts and Science, 2006).

13. Document reference no. D-3, Archive of the International Center for Unit 731 Research.

14. Document reference no. D-2, Archive of the International Center for Unit 731 Research.

Chapter 6

1. Doc. Title: AFPAC, CIC Report on Ishii, Dr. Shiro; Location: 270/84/16/05, RG#319, Entry#184B, Box 549, National Archives II of USA, Maryland.

2. Doc. Title: Ishii, Dr. Shiro; Location: 290/12/25/04, RG#331, Entry#1331, Box 1762, National Archives II of USA, Maryland.

3. Doc. Title: Lt-Gen. Ishii (Japanese Army Medical Corps); Location: 270/84/16/05, RG#319, Entry#184B, Box 549, National Archives II of USA, Maryland.

4. Doc. Title: 441st CIC Investigation on Whereabouts of Lt. Gen Shiro Ishii; Location:270/84/16/05, RG#319, Entry#184B, Box 549, National Archives II of USA, Maryland.

5. *Ibid.*

6. Doc. Title: GHQ, AFPAC Report on Whereabouts of Shiro Ishii; Location: 270/84/16/05, RG#319, Entry#184B, Box 549,National Archives II of USA, Maryland.

7. Doc. Title: GHQ, SCAP Letter to Central Liaison Office, Tokyo re Shiro Ishii; Location:270/84/16/05, RG#319, Entry#184B, Box 549, National Archives II of USA, Maryland.
8. Doc. Title: Biological Warfare Activities. Cover Sheet Transmitting Report; Location:270/84/16/05, G#319, Entry#184B, Box 549, National Archives II of USA, Maryland.
9. Doc. Title: 441st CIC Report Shiro Ishii has Failed to Report because He is Confined to Tokyo because of Illness; Location: 270/84/16/05, RG#319, Entry#184B, Box 549, National Archives II of USA, Maryland.
10. *Ibid.*
11. *Ibid.*
12. Doc. Title: Report on Scientific Intelligence Survey in Japan, September and October 1945. Volume 5, BIOLOGICAL WARFARE; Location: 2910, RG# IWG Ref. Coll., From GHQ, AFPAC, Scientific & Technical Advisory Sec; Author: Sanders, Murray & Young, Harry.
13. Doc Title: ISHII, Dr. Shiro; Location: 290/12/25/04, RG#331, ENTRY#1331, Box 1762, National Archives II of USA, Maryland.
14. Doc. Title: 441st CIC Report on Shiro Ishii; Location: 270/84/16/05, RG#319, Entry#184B, Box 549, National Archives II of USA, Maryland.
15. *Ibid.*
16. Doc. Title: Message C 52423. USSR Witnesses Kawashima & Karasawa Confirm Japanese BW Human Experiments, which Ishii characterises as 'Field Trials', Ishii Agrees to Describe BW Programme in Return for Immunity; Location: 290/24/02/03, RG#331, Entry#1901, Box 1, National Archives II of USA, Maryland.
17. Doc. Title: 441st CIC Report on Shiro Ishii; Location: 270/84/16/05, RG#319, Entry#184B, Box 549, National Archives II of USA, Maryland.
18. Doc. Title: Message W 98097. Replies to C52423 with 17 Questions on BW Field Experiments against Crops; Location: 290/24/02/03, RG#331, Entry#1901, Box 1, National Archives II of USA, Maryland.
19. Doc. Title: Brief Summary of New Information about Japanese BW Activities; Location: 290/03/19/02, RG#175, Entry#67A4900, Box196, National Archives II of USA, Maryland.
20. *Ibid.*
21. Doc. Title: Summary Report on B.W. Investigations; Location: 290/03/19/03, RG#175, Entry#67A4900, Box 217, National Archives II of USA, Maryland.
22. Doc. Title: Enclosure to SWNCC 351/D; Location: 270/02/13/07, RG#153, Entry#145, Box 73, National Archives II of USA, Maryland.
23. Doc. Title: Message W 94446. Instructions for prior US Interviews prior to any Russian Interrogations of Kikuchi, Ota, & Ishii; Location: 290/24/02/03, RG#331, Entry#1901, Box1, National Archives II of USA, Maryland.
24. *Ibid.*
25. Doc. Title: Message C 52423. USSR Witnesses Kawashima & Karasawa Confirm Japanese BW Human Experiments, which Ishii characterises as 'Field Trials', Ishii Agrees to Describe BW Programme in Return for Immunity; Location: 290/24/02/03, RG#331, Entry#1901, Box 1, National Archives II of USA, Maryland.
26. *Ibid.*
27. Doc. Title: Priority Action; War Crimes Branch, CAD; Location: 270/02/13/07, RG#153, Entry#145, Box 73, National Archives II of USA, Maryland.
28. Doc. Title: Message C 53169 Reply to W 99277; Location: 290/24/02/03, RG#331, Entry#1901, Box 1, National Archives II of USA, Maryland.
29. Doc. Title: Outgoing Classified Message; Location: 270/02/13/07, RG#153, Entry#145, Box 73, National Archives II of USA, Maryland.
30. Doc. Title: Message C 53663; Location: 290/24/02/03, RG#331, Entry#1901, Box 1, National Archives II of USA, Maryland.

31. Doc. Title: Outgoing Classified Message; Location: 270/02/13/07, RG#153, Entry#145, Box 73, National Archives II of USA, Maryland.

32. Sheldon H. Harris, *Factories of Death: Japanese Biological Warfare, 1932-1945, and the American cover-up* (New York: Routledge, 1996), p. 302.

33. Doc Title: Report on Scientific Intelligence Survey in Japan, September and October 1945. Volume 5, BIOLOGICAL WARFARE; Location: 2910, RG# IWG Ref. Coll. From GHQ, AFPAC, Scientific & Technical Advisory Sec; Author: Sanders, Murray & Young, Harry.

Epilogue

1. Kenneth L. Port, *Deciphering the History of Japanese War Atrocities: The Story of Doctor and General Shiro Ishii* (Durham, North Carolina: Carolina Academic Press, 2014), pp. ix.

2. Ecclesiastes 1:9.

Bibliography

'Brief Summary of New Information About Japanese BW Activities'; Location: 290/03/19/02, RG#175, ENTRY#67A4900, Box 196, National Archives II of USA.

A written material, Guanyu Shijing Budui de Jie Shao (Introduction to the Ishii Unit), submitted to the US military by Masaji Kitano the Commander of the Unit 731 on 1 April 1947. The document is now preserved at the National Archives II of USA, Maryland.

Archive of the Relief and Record Divison, Social Welfare and War Victims' Relief Bureau, Ministry of Health, Labour and Welfare, Japan.

Association of Returnees from China, *Qinlue: zaihua riben zhanfan de zhengyan* (*Invasion: Narrative from Japanese Criminals in China*) (China: Xintong Shushe, 2002).

Brief Summary of New Information About Japanese BW Activities; Location: 290/03/19/02, RG#175, ENTRY#67A4900, Box 196, National Archives II of USA.

Central Archives ed., *Riben Diguozhuyi Qinhua Dangan Ziliao Xuanbian: Xijunzhan yu Duqizhan* (*Selected Archival Records of the Japanese Imperialist's Invasion of China: Bacteriological Warfare and Poisonous Gas Warfare*) (Beijing: Zhonghua Book, 1989)

Chen Wengui, 'Report on plague in Changteh, Human', Report of the International Scientific Commission for the Investigation of the Facts Concerning Bacterial Warfare in Korea and China, (Beijing: 1952).

Chen Zhiyuan, Liu Yi, '12 Cases of Oral History Investigation of Victims of Bacteriological Warfare in Changteh', *Journal of Hunan University of Arts and Science*, vol. NO. 2006-03-10, (Changteh: Hunan University of Arts and Science, 2006).

Doc Title: 441st CIC Report on Shiro Ishii; Location: 270/84/16/05, RG#319, Entry#184B, Box 549, National Archives II of USA, Maryland.

Doc Title: Bacteriological Warfare; Location: 2910, RG#IWG Ref. Coll., Author: Masuda Tomosada. National Archives II of USA, Maryland.

Doc Title: Interrogation of Colonel Enryo HOJO; Location: 270/13/31/05, RG#319, ENTRY#85.

Doc Title: ISHII, Dr. Shiro; Location: 290/12/25/04, RG#331, ENTRY#1331, Box 1762, National Archives II of USA, Maryland.

Doc Title: Report on Scientific Intelligence Survey in Japan, September and October 1945. Volume 5, BIOLOGICAL WARFARE; Location: 2910, RG# IWG Ref. Coll. From GHQ, AFPAC, Scientific & Technical Advisory Sec; Author: Sanders, Murray & Young, Harry.

Doc Title: Summary Report on B.W. Investgations; Location: 290/03/19/03, RG#175, ENTRY#67A4900, Box 196, National Archives II of USA, Maryland.

Doc. Title: 441st CIC Investigation on Whereabouts of Lt. Gen Shiro Ishii; Location: 270/84/16/05, RG#319, Entry#184B, Box 549, National Archives II of USA, Maryland.

Doc. Title: 441st CIC Report Shiro Ishii has Failed to Report because He is Confined to Tokyo because of Illness; Location: 270/84/16/05, RG#319, Entry#184B, Box 549, National Archives II of USA, Maryland.

Doc. Title: AFPAC, CIC Report on Ishii, Dr. Shiro; Location: 270/84/16/05, RG#319, Entry#184B, Box 549, National Archives II of USA, Maryland.

Doc. Title: Biological Warfare Activities. Cover Sheet Transmitting Report; Location: 270/84/16/05, G#319, Entry#184B, Box 549, National Archives II of USA, Maryland.

Doc. Title: Brief Summary of New Information about Japanese BW Activities; Location: 290/03/19/02, RG#175, Entry#67A4900, Box 196, National Archives II of USA, Maryland.

Doc. Title: Enclosure to SWNCC 351/D; Location: 270/02/13/07, RG#153, Entry#145, Box 73, National Archives II of USA, Maryland.

Doc. Title: GHQ, AFPAC Report on Whereabouts of Shiro Ishii; Location: 270/84/16/05, RG#319, Entry#184B, Box 549,National Archives II of USA, Maryland.

Doc. Title: GHQ, SCAP Letter to Central Liaison Office, Tokyo re Shiro Ishii; Location: 270/84/16/05, RG#319, Entry#184B, Box 549, National Archives II of USA, Maryland.

Doc. Title: Ishii, Dr. Shiro; Location: 290/12/25/04, RG#331, Entry#1331, Box 1762, National Archives II of USA, Maryland.

Doc. Title: Lt-Gen. Ishii (Japanese Army Medical Corps); Location: 270/84/16/05, RG#319, Entry#184B, Box 549, National Archives II of USA, Maryland.

Doc. Title: Message C 52423. USSR Witnesses Kawashima & Karasawa Confirm Japanese BW Human Experiments, which Ishii characterises as 'Field Trials', Ishii Agrees to Describe BW Programme in Return for Immunity; Location: 290/24/02/03, RG#331, Entry#1901, Box 1, National Archives II of USA, Maryland.

Doc. Title: Message C 53169 Reply to W 99277; Location: 290/24/02/03, RG#331, Entry#1901, Box 1, National Archives II of USA, Maryland.

Doc. Title: Message C 53663; Location: 290/24/02/03, RG#331, Entry#1901, Box 1, National Archives II of USA, Maryland.

Doc. Title: Message W 94446. Instructions for prior US Interviews prior to any Russian Interrogations of Kikuchi, Ota, & Ishii; Location: 290/24/02/03, RG#331, Entry#1901, Box 1, National Archives II of USA, Maryland.

Doc. Title: Message W 98097. Replies to C52423 with 17 Questions on BW Field Experiments against Crops; Location: 290/24/02/03, RG#331, Entry#1901, Box 1, National Archives II of USA, Maryland.

Doc. Title: Outgoing Classified Message; Location:270/02/13/07, RG#153, Entry#145, Box73, National Archives II of USA, Maryland.

Doc. Title: Priority Action; War Crimes Branch, CAD; Location: 270/02/13/07, RG#153, Entry#145, Box 73, National Archives II of USA, Maryland.

Doc. Title: Report on Scientific Intelligence Survey in Japan, September and October 1945. Volume 5, BIOLOGICAL WARFARE; Location: 2910, RG# IWG Ref. Coll., From GHQ, AFPAC, Scientific & Technical Advisory Sec; Author: Sanders, Murray & Young, Harry.

Doc. Title: Summary Report on B.W. Investigations; Location: 290/03/19/03, RG#175, Entry#67A4900, Box 217, National Archives II of USA, Maryland.

Document no.: S11-10-42, Archive of Research Institute of Self-Defense of Japan, War Ministry.

Document reference no. D-2, Archive of the International Center for Unit 731 Research.

Document reference no. D-3, Archive of the International Center for Unit 731 Research.

Document reference no. E-1, Archive of the International Center for Unit 731 Research.

Document Reference no.: A-17. Archive of the Exhibition Hall of Evidences of Crime Committed by Unit 731 of the Japanese Imperial Army.

Document reference no.: B17-3, Archive of the International Center for Unit 731 Research.

Document reference no.: B-2, Archive of the International Center for Unit 731 Research.

Document Reference no.: C-121. Archive of the Exhibition Hall of Evidences of Crime Committed by Unit 731 of the Japanese Imperial Army.

Document reference no.: C-17, archive of the International Center for Unit 731 Research.

Document Reference no.: E-2. Archive of the Exhibition Hall of Evidences of Crime Committed by Unit 731 of the Japanese Imperial Army.

Document reference no.: E-21, Archive of the International Center for Unit 731 Research.

Ecclesiastes 1:9.

Fukiko Aoki, *Shijingsilang ji xijunzhan budui jie mi* (*The Secrets of Shirō Ishii and Biological Warfare Force*) (Shanghai: Shanghai Translation Publishing House, 2010).

Guo Sumei, *Renxing de Minmie yu Fusu* (*Obliteration and Revival of Human Nature*), read at the Seminar on Anti-invasion and Peace-keeping in Harbin in 1995.

Han Xiao and Xin Peilin, *Rijun Qisanyi Budui Zuieshi* (*Criminal History of the Unit 731 of the Japanese Military*) (Harbin: Heilongjiang People's Publishing House, 1991)

Hisato Yoshimura, *Memoir of My 77th Birthday*, (Kyoto: Aotian Yinshua Co., 1984).

Ichiro Kadowaki, 'Kyoto Medical College and Unit 731 of Japanese Kwantung Army,' *Journal of Research Society for 15 Years War and Japanese Medical Science and Service* 1 (2000).

Iwasaki Jirō, *Bukka no sesō 100nen* (*100 Years of the situation of commodity prices*). (Tokyo: Yomimura Shinbum Sha, 1982).

Ji Xueren ed., *Qinhua Rijun Duqizhan Shiliji* (*Examples of Poisonous Warfare by the Japan's China Expeditionary Army*) (Beijing: Social Sciences Academic Press, 2008).

Jin Chengmin, *Ribenjun Xijunzhan* (*Bacteriological Warfare of the Japanese Military*) (Harbin: Heilongjiang People's Publishing House, 2008).

Kenneth L. Port, *Deciphering the History of Japanese War Atrocities: The Story of Doctor and General Shiro Ishii* (Durham, North Carolina: Carolina Academic Press, 2014).

Matsumura Takao and Tanaka Akira ed., *15nen Senso Gokuhi Shiryōshū Dai 29 Shū Nanasanichi Butai Sakusei Shiryō* (Material written by the Unit 731) (Tokyo: Fujishuppan, 1991).

Miyatake Go, *Shōgun no Igen: Endō Sanrō no Nikki* (*General's Last Words: Diary of Endō Sanrō*) (Tokyo: The Mainichi Newspaper Co., 1986).

Morimura Seiichi, Zu Binghe tran., *Shiren Moku: Riben Guandongjun Xijunzhan Budui de Kongbu Neimu* (*Ogre's Cave: Terrible Inside Story of the Bacteriological Warfare Unit from Japan's Kwantung Army*) (Beijing: Qunzhong Chubanshe, 1984).

NA, RG38, BOX2097: A report by Lt-Col. Arvo T. Thompson, V.C, Army Service Forces, Camp Detrick. Maryland. Report on Japanese Biological Warfare(BW) Activities May 31, 1946.

Naval Aspects of Biological Warfare; Author: Inglis, RADM Thomas B.; Location: 190/25/17/07, RG#330, ENTRY#199, Box 103, National Archives II of USA.

No. 78 operation order issued by the Kanto Army Command kept at the Japanese National Archives of Official Documents.

Qianriben Lujun Junren Yinzhunbei he Shiyong Xijun Wuqi Beikongan Shenpan Cailiao (*Trial Material of the Case that Former Japanese Army Prepared and Used Bacteriological Weapons*), (Moscow: Waiguo Wenshuji Chubanju, 1950).

Report on Japanese Biological Warfare (BW) Activities; Location: 2910, RG#IWG Ref. Coll, National Archives II of USA.

Sadao Koshi, *Hinomaru ha akai namida ni* (*Bloody Tears on Hinomaru*) (Japan: Kyoiku Shiryo Shuppankai, 1983).

Sheldon H. Harris, *Factories of Death: Japanese Biological Warfare, 1932–1945 and The American Cover-up*, (Routlege: 1996).

Shozo Azami, 'The Medical Crime in the Fifteen Years' War and Our Task Today', *Journal of Research Society for 15 years War and Japanese Medical Science and Service*, vol. 12, (Japan: Research Society for 15 years War and Japanese Medical Science and Service, 2011).

Shuli Ji, *Shuyi* (*Plague*) (Beijing: People's Medical Publishing House Co. Ltd, 2010).

Study Group of Hygiene Research in Winter, Gokuhi Chūmōgun Tōki Eisei Kenkyū Seiseki (Tokyo: Gendai Shokan, 1941).

The School of Army Surgeon ed., *Rikkun Kuni Gakkō Gojūnen Shi* (*50 Years of History of the School of Army Surgeon*) (Tokyo: Fujishuppan, 1988).

United Nations Office for Disarmament Affairs, disarmament.un.org/treaties/t/bwc/text, accessed on 21 June 2016.

United Nations Office for Disarmament Affairs, unoda-web.s3-accelerate.amazonaws.com/wp-content/uploads/assets/WMD/Bio/pdf/Status_Protocol.pdf, accessed on 21 June 2016.

Video document reference no.: A18-8, Archive of the International Center for Unit 731 Research.

Video document reference no.: B-3, Archive of the International Center for Unit 731 Research.

Video document reference no.: B-3, Archive of the International Center for Unit 731 Research.

War and Medicine, an exhibition panel brochure prepared by The Research Society for 15 Years' War and Japanese Medical Science and Service, (Japan: Sanhuishe, 2006), p. 1.